ALZHEIMER'S DISEASE

A Handbook for Caregivers

ALZHEIMER'S DISEASE
A Handbook for Caregivers

RONALD C. HAMDY, MD, FRCP

Professor of Medicine,
Associate Chief of Staff/Extended Care and Geriatrics,
Veterans Administration Medical Center;
Chief, Division of Geriatric Medicine,
James H. Quillen College of Medicine,
East Tennessee State University,
Johnson City, Tennessee;
President, Northeast Tennessee
Chapter, Alzheimer's Association

JAMES M. TURNBULL, MD, FRCP(C)

Staff Psychiatrist, Holston Mental Health Services,
Kingsport Tennessee; Clinical Professor of Psychiatry,
James H. Quillen College of Medicine,
East Tennessee State University,
Johnson City, Tennessee

LINDA D. NORMAN, RN, MSN

Director, Nursing Program, Aquinas Junior College,
Nashville, Tennessee

MARY M. LANCASTER, RNC, MSN

Clinical Nurse Specialist—Gerontology,
Veterans Administration Medical Center,
Mountain Home, Tennessee;
Consultant, Center for Geriatrics and Gerontology;
Adjunct Clinical Instructor, School of Nursing,
East Tennessee State University,
Johnson City, Tennessee

The C. V. Mosby Company

ST. LOUIS · BALTIMORE · PHILADELPHIA · TORONTO   1990

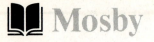 **Mosby**

Editor: Linda L. Duncan
Editorial Assistant: Rebecca Sweeney
Project Manager: Patricia Gayle May
Designer: Gail Morey Hudson

FIRST EDITION

Printed in the United States of America

The C.V. Mosby Company
11830 Westline Industrial Drive, St. Louis, Missouri, 63146

Library of Congress Cataloging in Publication Data

Alzheimer's disease : a handbook for caregivers / Ronald C. Hamdy . . .
  [et al.]. — 1st ed.
    p.   cm.
  Includes bibliographical references.
  ISBN 0-8016-2026-0
  1. Alzheimer's disease. 2. Alzheimer's disease—Complications and
sequelae. 3. Alzheimer's disease—Family relationships.
  4. Alzheimer's disease—Social aspects.   I. Hamdy, R. C.
RC523.A386   1990
618.97′6831—dc20   90-5682
                                                             CIP

GW/D/D 9 8 7 6 5 4 3 2 1

7-23-90

Contributors

BEA ABERNATHY, RN

Founder and Chairman, Alzheimer's Research,
Care and Educational Center, Upper East Tennessee,
Kingsport, Tennessee

ROBERT V. ACUFF, PhD

Director, Division of Clinical Nutrition,
Department of Surgery, James H. Quillen College of Medicine,
East Tennessee State University,
Johnson City, Tennessee

JOYCE BROOME, RN

Nurse Practitioner, Nursing Home Care Unit,
Veterans Administration Medical Center,
Mountain Home, Tennessee

PATRICIA S. BROWN

Director, First Tennessee Area Agency on Aging,
Johnson City, Tennessee

ROBERTA "MICKEY" GROSSMAN

Consultant, Occupational Therapist, Northside Hospital,
Johnson City, Tennessee

RONALD C. HAMDY, MD, FRCP

Professor of Medicine,
Associate Chief of Staff/Extended Care and Geriatrics,
Veterans Administration Medical Center;
Chief, Division of Geriatric Medicine,
James H. Quillen College of Medicine,
East Tennessee State University,
Johnson City, Tennessee;
President, Northeast Tennessee
Chapter, Alzheimer's Association

MARY McLEOD LANCASTER, RNC, MSN

Clinical Nurse Specialist—Gerontology,
Veterans Administration Medical Center,
Mountain Home, Tennessee;
Consultant, Center for Geriatrics and Gerontology;
Adjunct Clinical Instructor,
School of Nursing,
East Tennessee State University,
Johnson City, Tennessee

KENNETH MATHEWS Jr., MD, MSPH

Health Officer, Sullivan County Health Department,
Tennessee Department of Health and Environment;
Clinical Assistant Professor,
Department of Internal Medicine,
James H. Quillen College of Medicine,
East Tennessee State University,
Johnson City, Tennessee

MARGUERITE METTETAL

Public Guardian for the Elderly,
First Tennessee Area Agency on Aging,
Johnson City, Tennessee

LINDA D. NORMAN, RN, MSN

Director, Nursing Program, Aquinas Junior College,
Nashville, Tennessee

EDITH PATRICK

Caregiver,
Johnson City, Tennessee

PATRICK SLOAN, PhD

Clinical Psychologist, Veterans Administration Medical Center;
Clinical Associate Professor, Department of Psychiatry and
Behavioral Sciences, Department of Internal Medicine,
James H. Quillen College of Medicine,
East Tennessee State University,
Johnson City, Tennessee

ELIZABETH H. SMITH, PhD, RN

Associate Professor and Coordinator of Research,
School of Nursing, East Tennessee State University,
Johnson City, Tennessee

JAMES M. TURNBULL, MD, FRCP(C)

Staff Psychiatrist,
Holston Mental Health Services,
Kingsport, Tennessee;
Clinical Professor of Psychiatry,
James H. Quillen College of Medicine,
East Tennessee State University,
Johnson City, Tennessee

SHARON TURNBULL, RN, PhD

Director, Center for Adult Programs and Services,
Clinical Associate Professor of Family Practice,
East Tennessee State University,
Johnson City, Tennessee

WILLIAM G. WOOD, PhD, MD

Medical Director, Woodridge Hospital;
Clinical Associate Professor,
Department of Psychiatry,
James H. Quillen College of Medicine,
East Tennessee State University,
Johnson City, Tennessee

To
our patients with Alzheimer's disease
and to
their relatives and caregivers
from whom we have learned and continue to learn so much.

Foreword

The full tragedy of Alzheimer's disease, which affects one out of every ten Americans over the age of 65, was impressed upon me during a series of Congressional hearings I chaired in 1984. At a hearing in Tennessee, a woman whose husband suffers from Alzheimer's offered testimony I will never forget. "A few months ago," she began, "my husband asked me to go into the bedroom — we needed to talk privately, he said. I went to the room and closed the door. Turning to me with tears in his eyes he asked, 'Am I losing my mind, honey? Am I going crazy?'" She went on: "My life can be described as a funeral that never ends . . . I want my husband back."

That woman is not alone. Two to three million "never-ending funerals" are sapping the strength of both victims and their families across America. A concerted effort is long overdue to defeat this disease which erodes the mental and physical health of the patient before his or her time. Part of the solution lies in research to uncover the causes of the disease and develop treatments for it. Just as crucial, however, is assuring that those who take care of patients with Alzheimer's know as much about the problem as possible.

That is one reason I am so pleased with *Alzheimer's Disease: A Handbook for Caregivers*, which contains a wealth of practical information about the effects of Alzheimer's on the patient's day-to-day life. The book offers detailed descriptions of the stages of the disease, the options for treatment, and the effects of other mental and physical characteristics upon the expression of Alzheimer's. It also offers valuable suggestions for approaching issues such as nutrition, sleep habits, and therapy. The book is a perfect bridge between those who know most about the disease — and those who know most about the patient.

Congress, by establishing regional centers devoted to the research and treatment of Alzheimer's, has taken one step in the right direction. The medical faculty at East Tennessee State University, by creating this fine book, has taken another. Perhaps, through more efforts like these, we can begin to lift some of the fear and uncertainty that surround this national tragedy.

Albert Gore, Jr.
U.S. Senator

Preface

Alzheimer's disease has been called "the disease of the century." It afflicts up to three million Americans, mostly people over the age of 65. It may be the harshest of all the incurable diseases because, in a way, it hits its victims twice. First, the mind dies, with the simplest tasks such as eating with a knife and fork, telling time, or putting on a dress, becoming insurmountable. Second, the body dies. Victims become unable to walk or control their body functions. In the end the victim lies curled in a fetal position gradually sinking into coma and death.

Alzheimer's disease is even more devastating for the families and caregivers of its victims. The caregivers drive themselves to physical and emotional exhaustion while they render continuous care and experience the anguish of seeing a loved one turned into a person who no longer remembers who he or she is.

While researchers struggle to understand the disease and look for drugs that will slow its progress, it is becoming increasingly clear that patients with Alzheimer's disease are not beyond help. In the early stages of the disease, aids to memory, behavior therapy, day care centers, respite care, and some simple understanding of how the disease works can postpone the day when the victim must be placed in a nursing home.

This book was written in response to a request from caregivers in our community—individuals who care for victims at home and health care professionals who look after patients in nursing homes. We recognized the need for a comprehensive book that would address many of the issues faced by caregivers who are expected to help the victims of this devastating illness. Although the disease affects more women than men, we have chosen to use the male pronoun throughout the text. It is

hoped that this book will prove of real value to those who are expected
to care for this growing population of individuals with what has to date
been an incurable disease.

Ronald C. Hamdy
James M. Turnbull
Linda D. Norman
Mary M. Lancaster

Acknowledgments

We would like to thank all our colleagues who have referred to us patients suffering from dementing illnesses and Alzheimer's disease, thus allowing us to gain a wider experience in this field. We also would like to thank the patients' relatives and caregivers who have given us so much information and insight on the illness and its impact on their lives. We also wish to thank Christine O'Neil for editing the final version of the manuscript and the staff of the C. V. Mosby Company for their work on this book. Finally, we would like to thank Ms. Kathy Whalen and Ms. Janice Lyons for their painstaking secretarial work and efficient help in producing this manuscript.

Contents

ALZHEIMER'S DISEASE: THE PROBLEM

1
Clinical presentation

R. Hamdy

In 1907 Dr. Alois Alzheimer described one of the first cases of the disease that now bears his name. Dr. Alzheimer, a physician in a German asylum, had noticed that one woman's condition seemed quite different from that of most of the other patients.

The woman was only 51 years old. Her main problems were a very poor memory and a tendency to get lost in the asylum. She was not violent or aggressive, but she had to be confined because she was unable to look after herself. Dr. Alzheimer noted that she had some language impairment, including difficulty finding the right words, and that her comprehension was impaired. When he examined the patient, Dr. Alzheimer could not identify any neurological deficit. Her motor power was good, sensations were normal, and all the tendon reflexes were present and within normal limits. Her gait and coordination were unremarkable.

Dr. Alzheimer followed up on the patient for about 4½ years, until she died after a gradual but relentless deterioration. He performed a postmortem examination and found that her brain was much smaller than the average brain of people of the same sex and age. He also noticed that the ventricles (cavities normally present in the brain) were dilated and much larger than he had expected. It was as if the brain had shrunk and atrophied. A microscopic examination revealed a reduced number of brain cells and numerous neurofibrillary tangles and senile plaques. All these findings comprise the characteristic features of Alzheimer's disease.

AGE OF ONSET

Probably because the first patient to be reported was only 51 years old and because the next few cases to be described were also in patients

3

under 65 years of age, the general assumption formerly was that Alzheimer's disease affected predominantly younger people. At the turn of the century, it was thought that mental functions tended to deteriorate as an individual aged. Thus different terms were needed to distinguish the impairment of mental functions that occurs in old age ("senile dementia") from that which occurs in younger people, and the term "presenile dementia" was introduced. A few cases of the disease manifesting itself in the fourth decade were reported, and these reinforced the concept that Alzheimer's disease should be classified as a "presenile dementia." Indeed, until fairly recently the diagnosis of Alzheimer's disease was restricted to patients under 65 years of age.

However, as clinical and postmortem findings resulted in more cases being described in patients over 65 years of age, it was acknowledged that Alzheimer's disease was not confined to young people but that it also was seen in older patients. Thus yet another term was introduced: senile dementia of the Alzheimer's type (SDAT).

For some time the debate went on as to whether Alzheimer's disease affecting younger people (presenile dementia) was the same condition as senile dementia of the Alzheimer's type. Some raised the question of whether the disorder was one disease that could have an early onset (presenile dementia) and a late onset (senile dementia), or whether there were basically two different diseases that sometimes displayed the same or similar features.

Only recently was a consensus reached, and it now is generally accepted that the presenile and senile types of Alzheimer's disease are the same. The tendency now is to refer to Alzheimer's disease and to note that its onset can occur early or late in life.

The two forms of the disease, early onset and late onset, must be differentiated, because when Alzheimer's disease starts early in life, the prognosis often is poor. In general, the earlier the disease manifests itself, the more severe it is and the quicker is the rate of deterioration. Conversely, when Alzheimer's disease manifests itself later in life, it frequently is much less severe and the rate of deterioration usually is very slow. There is, however, a wide range of variation among patients.

FAMILIAL TENDENCY

When the disease manifests itself at an early age, the familial tendency is more marked than if it starts at a later age. Therefore the chances of the patient's children developing the disease are higher if their parents developed it at an early age. Interestingly, "familial" Alzheimer's disease tends to affect both sexes equally, whereas Alzheimer's disease that occurs in old age tends to affect women slightly more frequently than men.

The past few years have seen considerable progress in the study of the genes of patients with Alzheimer's disease, and defects in chromosome 21 (the same chromosome that is abnormal in Down's syndrome) have been identified. Genetic markers also may be present in Alzheimer's disease. These studies are still at the experimental level and currently have no practical applications. However, in the future, studying the genetic pattern may enable researchers to identify people likely to develop the disease at a later stage.

CLINICAL SYMPTOMS
Memory Deficit

Memory usually is divided into three different forms: immediate memory (remembering for a few seconds), short-term memory (remembering for a few minutes or hours), and long-term memory (remembering for a few years). Early in Alzheimer's disease, the short-term memory is impaired but some long-term memory is preserved. Immediate memory is also affected, but this is probably secondary to a short attention span. The main problem for patients with Alzheimer's disease is the short-term memory impairment, which interferes with social and professional activities. However, this memory impairment must be differentiated from that sometimes seen in normal people, which is often called "benign forgetfulness."

The main difference between memory impairment in Alzheimer's disease and benign forgetfulness is that the former is undiscriminating and constant and interferes with the patient's social and professional activities. Benign forgetfulness, on the other hand, usually is sporadic, limited to trivial matters, and does not significantly interfere with the patient's life, apart from causing frustration and irritation, as when a person cannot remember where the keys were left. Unlike the memory impairment associated with Alzheimer's disease, that seen in benign forgetfulness usually can be remedied fairly easily, for example, by concentrating and trying to remember or by keeping written records. In Alzheimer's disease, although patients initially may try to overcome their problem by writing down what they want to remember, sooner or later the memory deficit is such that they may forget to check their written record.

Obviously, the degree of impairment necessary to interfere with a patient's social and professional life depends a great deal on the person's activities. This may best be demonstrated by comparing two patients of the same age, a housewife and a pharmacist. The housewife lives with her husband and is dependent on him, since she has been crippled with osteoarthritis for a number of years. She does not have to pay bills or shop. She does some cooking, but her husband by and large makes most of the decisions and does most of the housework. By the time her memory impairment affects her day-to-day activities, it will have to be quite severe.

Any degree of memory deficit experienced by the pharmacist would interfere with her professional life. She may not be able to remember the names of the drugs or the dosage on the prescriptions she has to dispense. Therefore, even though the degree of mental impairment may be mild, it is constant and sufficient to interfere with the patient's professional life and thus must be considered part of a dementing process rather than benign forgetfulness. Whether this dementing process is secondary to Alzheimer's disease depends on the rest of the patient's clinical picture and laboratory investigations. To summarize, the extent of mental impairment necessary to interfere with a person's social and professional activities depends on the person's profession and daily activities.

Early in the course of the disease, patients usually are aware of their memory deficit and they may make notes to remember important things. Often they also become frightened and apprehensive about their memory problems and may become depressed and discouraged. As the disease progresses, patients lose insight into their memory deficit and no longer are aware of it. At this point patients must be "protected from themselves." For instance, they may try to prepare a meal and forget the stove is on or may try to drive, oblivious to the fact that they are becoming lost or are making dangerous errors in judgment.

Inability to Acquire New Knowledge Information

One of the earliest manifestations of Alzheimer's disease is an inability to acquire and retain new information and to integrate it with previously acquired knowledge. This is partly the result of short-term memory impairment and can be readily observed in the difficulty the patient has in keeping abreast of recent developments in his profession and an inability to discuss current events. These difficulties often lead the patient to withdraw from discussions revolving around these topics, and he may appear to have lost interest in these particular fields.

Not infrequently the first indication that something is wrong occurs when the patient has to learn something new at work. For instance, computerization is introduced in the office or the patient's job is reorganized. He may be unable to adapt to these changes, and consequently his colleagues may think that he is "getting old" and set in his ways. At this stage the patient may elect to take early retirement or may be assigned a more routine, less demanding job.

Alternatively, a sudden change in a person's environment may trigger an episode of severe confusion in which he suddenly finds himself in a strange place and is unable to remember how he got there. For instance, during a stay in a hotel or a visit with his children, he may wake up in the middle of the night and be disoriented in space and time and grossly confused. He also may become agitated. In the early stages of Alzheimer's disease, this state does not last long. With explanation and reassurance, the patient soon becomes reoriented, alert, and "rational."

Language Difficulties

Anomia, the inability to find the right word, and agnosia, the inability to recognize and name objects, are characteristic features of Alzheimer's disease, even in the early stages when they may be so subtle that most people do not notice the impairment and only meticulous psychological testing can identify these deficits. (These tests are described in the section dealing with neuropsychological testing.) In the early stages the patient usually is aware of these deficits and may try to make up for them by using sentences to describe the object he cannot name (paraphrasia). Thus in the very early stages of Alzheimer's disease, the patient's speech may seem quite picturesque and interesting. In fact, the patient is only trying hard to overcome the problems of anomia and agnosia.

As the disease progresses, the agnosia becomes more extensive and the patient cannot use sensory information to recognize objects or people. As a result patients cannot recognize their spouses and other relatives and often accuse them of being intruders. As time goes by, the anomia also becomes quite marked, and the paraphrasia becomes less related to the target word and more rambling. At this stage conversation becomes very difficult. This situation is worsened by the patient's inability either to concentrate for any length of time or to comprehend spoken (and written) language. Not infrequently words and themes related to previous discussions and unrelated to the present conversation tend to intrude. As a result the listener is unable to follow any coherent train of thought.

Aphasia, an impairment in language, prevents the patient from understanding what he hears, from following instructions, and from communicating needs such as the need to go to the toilet or being in pain. This is distressing to the patient and trying to the caregivers, who now must guess what the patient's needs are. As the disease progresses, spontaneous speech deteriorates. The patient tends to repeat words and questions (echolalia) without making any effort to answer the questions. With further deterioration the patient repeats the same word (paralalia) or the first syllable of a word (logoclonia) over and over. In the advanced stage of the disease speech becomes unintelligible, and eventually complete mutism sets in.

Impaired Visuospatial Skills and Apraxia

Apraxia, an inability to carry out purposeful movements and actions despite intact motor and sensory systems, is evident early in the course of Alzheimer's disease, but patients and relatives often do not connect it with the disease. In the early stages, for instance, a patient may be unable to tie a bow tie but still be able to tie a regular tie, and he may attribute his inability to tie the former to "lack of practice." In fact, it represents an early stage of apraxia.

Apraxia often becomes a source of frustration: Minor tasks the patient used to perform easily become major tasks with almost insurmountable obstacles. The patient does not understand what is happening or how or why he is losing control over his environment. This often leads to discouragement and depression. As the disease progresses, even simple tasks become difficult. For instance, when asked to set the table, the patient is faced with so many choices (knives, forks, spoons, plates, glasses) and so many alternative positions for the items that he may not be able to tackle this "complex" task. On the other hand, if given only a knife, a fork, and a plate, he may be able to deal with this limited choice and arrange them adequately on the table.

In later stages the patient may be unable to adjust simultaneously the controls of the video recorder and the television set, although he may still be able to adjust each independently. In other words, the more complex or technical skills, particularly those recently acquired or requiring integration of various stimuli, are lost early in the process. The "automatic" actions such as eating, walking, dressing, and undressing tend to be preserved until late stages. This discrepancy exists because the complex and technical skills are controlled mostly by the cerebral cortex, and the automatic actions are controlled by the basal ganglia (this relationship is discussed further in Chapter 23.)

Impaired visuospatial skills may be the reason a patient becomes lost in familiar surroundings or while driving a car. In the latter instance, however, the inability to integrate new information and to make rational decisions also plays an important part.

As the disease progresses, even getting dressed becomes an impossible task. The patient may see his shirt and recognize the front, back, and left and right sides, but he is unable to translate these stimuli and coordinate his movements accordingly to put the right sleeve of his shirt on his right arm while keeping the top part of the shirt up and its front on his chest.

Poor Judgment

Sooner or later the patient's ability to use correct judgment also deteriorates. This may be the point at which relatives recognize the disease. They no longer consider the person odd or eccentric but realize that something is seriously wrong. This point often is reached when the patient pays the same bill twice or does not pay some bills or cannot balance the checkbook. Difficulty in managing finances is one of the commonest reasons relatives insist that a person seek medical attention.

Poor judgment may also be reflected by large donations to charity made after the patient has watched a television advertisement by a charitable organization or after he has spoken to unscrupulous representatives who take advantage of the person's impaired ability to make rational decisions. Sometimes the patient may start buying unnecessary items or extravagant gifts.

Self-Neglect

Another degree of mental impairment is reached when, in addition to impaired memory and impaired judgment, the patient shows evidence of carelessness, particularly self-neglect. One of the earliest manifestations is that patients stop taking pride in the impression they make. This is a very useful sign, especially for a woman patient, and can be appreciated by looking at her general appearance. For instance, if she makes no attempt to comb her hair and if her dress is stained or torn, in the absence of physical incapacitation, self neglect can be assumed.

In hospitals and nursing homes this carelessness and self-neglect can be easily appreciated by asking the patient to get up from her chair and to take a few steps. If after standing up she adjusts her clothes before walking or makes sure that her hospital gown is properly closed and that none of her private parts are exposed, then she obviously is aware of her body image and cares about the impression she projects in public. A patient with Alzheimer's disease, when asked to stand up and walk, may do so without realizing that the hospital gown is wide open from the back. She also would probably walk the length of the room without making any effort to cover her back and without showing signs of embarrassment; in fact, she is not aware of and does not care about the image she projects in public.

Behavioral Problems

Aberrant behavior is almost always distressing to both caregivers and patients. Such behavior may include stubbornness, resistance to care, suspicion of others, use of abusive language, acting upon delusions or hallucinations, rummaging through other people's rooms, "stealing," hiding articles, urinating in inappropriate places, and angry outbursts (sometimes called "catastrophic reactions") precipitated by apparently trivial events.

These abnormal behavioral patterns often are the reason caregivers seek institutionalization for the patient. Ironically, these same behaviors frequently are the reason nursing homes refuse to admit patients with Alzheimer's disease, on the grounds that such behavior would disrupt the harmony of the institution, may be offensive and dangerous to other residents, and may lead to litigation. Because of this aberrant behavior, patients often are prescribed potent sedatives and tranquilizers and are physically restrained.

Restlessness, aimless wandering, and reversal of the sleep/wake cycle are often seen in patients with Alzheimer's disease and frequently put the patient at risk of injuring himself.

Patients with Alzheimer's disease sometimes engage in asocial sexual behavior, such as masturbating in front of others. Although such practices are distressing to caregivers, especially the patient's children, there is no evidence to suggest that patients with dementia pose a sexual threat to others. (This is discussed further in Chapter 8.)

Physical Deterioration

Most patients with Alzheimer's disease remain physically well until the late stages of the disease, when they develop generalized muscle rigidity and later become bedridden and incontinent of urine and feces.

The three most common causes of death are pneumonia, urinary tract infection, and decubiti.

Clinical stages

Regardless of how the three stages of Alzheimer's disease are delineated, it is important to realize that they have been arbitrarily defined and that they overlap a great deal. Also, it must be emphasized that the time frame for each stage is not absolute, because patients do not deteriorate at the same rate nor do all necessarily go through the three stages. And, as mentioned previously, the earlier the disease manifests itself, the quicker is its progression and the worse the prognosis.

It is also important to realize that Alzheimer's disease has a very insidious onset and a slow, relentless progress. One of the best indicators of these two aspects of the disease is the relatives' inability to agree on a specific date when the symptoms started to manifest themselves. For instance, the daughter may think it was last Christmas, whereas the son-in-law may think that the patient's condition started to deteriorate well before this. In contrast to strokes or multiinfarct dementia, nobody can pinpoint an exact date or time when the disease manifested itself or the patient's condition suddenly deteriorated.

Stage 1

Stage 1 lasts between 1 and 3 years and is characterized by the following:

Poor recent memory
Impaired acquisition of new information
Mild anomia
Minimal visuospatial impairment
Personality change

This is a difficult period, because the patient still has some insight into his condition and yet cannot understand or cope with the complexity of his situation. At times the patient may "rebel" and refuse to accept the implications of his condition; at other times he may realize that he is fighting a losing battle and become depressed and irritable or withdraw into apathy.

This stage can also be particularly taxing for the patient's family. On one hand, they understand and appreciate the patient's actions; on the other hand, they question the validity of his judgment and yet do not want to appear to question or doubt his integrity, intentions, and ability to look after his family. This situation may require professional intervention to safeguard the family's financial assets.

A particularly difficult decision concerns the patient's ability to drive a motor vehicle. Driving is a symbol of independence and may be the person's only means of transportation. However, while driving the patient may make serious mistakes that could endanger himself or others. In addition to having poor judgment, many patients with Alzheimer's disease may have a slow reaction time and may be easily distracted, making driving hazardous.

Toward the end of stage 1, memory impairment and impaired ability to make rational decisions often cause the patient to become lost even in familiar surroundings. This is another traumatic and stressful experience for the patient's relatives. For example, a husband goes to a store in the next block to buy something and 2 hours later has not returned. Five hours later the police call the wife to tell her that they have found her husband in a place a few miles away.

Understandably, a patient's relatives may be reluctant to take away his sense of initiative and independence by confining him indoors. Yet, whenever he leaves home, they worry that he may become lost, be mugged, or be involved in an accident. Often the relatives resort to writing their address and phone number on a card and leaving it in one of the patient's pockets.

Patients with Alzheimer's disease become lost because they may not recognize familiar signs; they then do not know where they are and start to panic. When they panic, their judgment becomes even worse, and they may not be able to retrace their steps. Whereas stress may sharpen a normal person's mental abilities, in a patient with dementia it may lead to severe confusion.

In the first stage the clinical examination is essentially within normal limits, although some patients have a reduced sense of smell. The computerized tomography (CT) scan and electroencephalogram (EEG) are usually essentially normal, as are the other tests that may be done routinely.

Stage 2

Stage 2 lasts between 2 and 10 years and is characterized by the following:

Profound memory loss, remote as well as recent

Significant impairment of other cognitive parameters, as evidenced by two or more of these symptoms: anomia, agnosia, apraxia, and aphasia

Severe loss of judgment

It is diagnostically important to make sure that the patient has these deficits. If they are absent, the dementia may not be Alzheimer's disease but rather a different type of dementia (e.g., multiinfarct dementia or the so-called subcortical dementias such as in Parkinson's disease) that may respond to treatment.

In the second stage the anomia and agnosia become much more pronounced and interfere with the patient's activities. Later in this stage the patient may develop significant apraxia, leaving him unable to perform simple tasks such as feeding or washing himself even though he has no muscle weakness or coordination difficulties.

In the second stage, patients with Alzheimer's disease tend to become very restless; they often are seen pacing the room or walking outside as if constantly searching for something. They do not like to stay in one place and want to keep moving.

The patient's personality, which in the first stage was variable, now is mostly apathetic. He has no insight into his condition and does not seem bothered by his relatives' distress over it.

This lack of insight is exemplified by the patient's denial of problems with his memory, despite evidence of profound memory loss. If confronted with the fact that his memory is poor, he usually makes some excuse, such as that he was not really paying attention, or that he is getting old, or that he has other things to remember and could not be bothered with such details.

The patient may make "near misses" when asked which day of the week it is; he may say that today is Monday rather than Tuesday. When corrected, he may question the relevance of today being Tuesday rather than Monday. If an examiner asks him to remember three or four objects, he may question the importance of being able to do so. In contrast, patients suffering from depression readily acknowledge problems with their memory, and rather than making "near misses," they refuse to cooperate with an examiner.

In stage 2, a CT scan usually shows evidence of brain atrophy and ventricular dilation. The EEG also may be abnormal.

Stage 3

Stage 3 lasts between 8 and 12 years and is characterized by the following:

Severe impairment of all cognitive functions

Physical impairment

Total loss of ability to care for oneself

Gross intellectual impairment is very obvious at this stage. For example, a patient may not even be able to recognize his wife and children and may often confuse them with his parents. Complete disorientation to time, place, and other individuals is evident, and the patient cannot look after even his basic needs. As the condition progresses, complete mutism may occur and motor deficits may become apparent; the patient may develop generalized muscular rigidity, and his mobility may be grossly reduced.

In contrast to the second stage, in which the patient wandered constantly, he now spends most of the time sitting in a chair or lying in bed. An attitude of generalized flexion gradually is adopted, with the patient lying curled up in bed. At this stage urinary and sometimes fecal incontinence may develop.

The CT scan shows gross atrophy and ventricular dilation, and the EEG shows slow waves.

Staging of a Patient

In general, stages proceed thus: In the first stage, memory is impaired; in the second stage, there is in addition evidence of gross deficits in other cognitive fields; in the third stage, besides the severe intellectual deterioration, physical deficits become apparent.

In the first stage all clinical investigations are essentially normal, including the CT scan and the EEG. In the second and third stages they usually are abnormal.

CAUSE OF DEATH

The usual cause of death is not Alzheimer's disease itself but rather aspiration pneumonia, urinary tract infection, or decubiti with septicemia. Decubiti are very likely to develop unless pressure areas are given special care.

Although Alzheimer's disease is characteristically irreversible and slowly progressive, it often is punctuated by sudden bouts of reversible deterioration caused by other diseases or factors apart from Alzheimer's disease. These are discussed in Chapter 3.

BIBLIOGRAPHY

Berg L et al: Mild senile dementia of the Alzheimer type: 2. Longitudinal assessment, Ann Neurol 23(5):477-484, 1988.

Folstein MF and Whitehouse PJ: Cognitive impairment of Alzheimer disease, Neurobehav Toxicol Teratol (6):631-634, 1983.

Hamill RW et al: Neurodegenerative disorders and aging. Alzheimer's disease and Parkinson's disease—common ground, Ann NY Acad Sci 515:411-420, 1988.

Katzman R: Alzheimer's disease, N Engl J Med 314(15):964-973, 1986.

Mohs RC, Rosen WG, and Davis KL: The Alzheimer's disease assessment scale: an instrument for assessing treatment efficacy, Psychopharmacol Bull 19(3):448-450, 1983.

Ninos M and Makohon R: Alzheimer's disease. Functional assessment of the patient, Geriatr Nurs 6(3):139-142, 1985.

Rathmann KL and Conner CS: Alzheimer's disease: clinical features, pathogenesis, and treatment, Drug Intell Clin Pharm 18(9):684-691, 1984.

Rosen WG: Clinical and neuropsychological assessment of Alzheimer disease, Adv Neurol 38:51-64, 1983.

Shapiro S, Hamby CL and Shapiro DL: Alzheimer's disease: an emerging affliction of the aging population, J Am Dent Assoc 111(2):287-292, 1985.

Winogrond IR and Fisk AA: Alzheimer's disease: assessment of functional status, J Am Geriatr Soc 31(12):780-785, 1983.

2

Diagnosis of Alzheimer's disease

J. Turnbull

The diagnosis of Alzheimer's disease is one of exclusion, because other diseases with a similar clinical picture must be ruled out. One such disease, for example, is delirium, an acute medical condition with symptoms of disorientation, confusion, and fluctuating levels of consciousness. Unlike Alzheimer's disease, delirum has a rapid onset and frequently is reversible when the underlying condition is corrected. Alzheimer's disease is not characterized by fluctuating levels of consciousness, at least not in the early stages.

The easiest, earliest, and most important part of the patient evaluation is the history, which is obtained not only from the individual but also from the relatives. Of particular interest, of course, is how long the process has been going on and what sort of behavior the patient has been demonstrating that indicates to the relatives that he is confused and amnesic. The differential diagnosis can be memorized by the mnemonic DEMENTIA, which is easy to remember because Alzheimer's disease is one of the two major dementias (the other being multiinfarct dementia).

"D" IS FOR DRUGS AND ALCOHOL

When evaluating a person who is confused and suffering from memory loss, the first thing that should be considered is drugs that the individual is taking. One drug that frequently is overlooked in the elderly is alcohol. A significant number of people, particularly men, become alcoholic after they retire. They may have been drinkers who had stopped drinking because they were afraid they would not be able to get to work the next day. Or they may have drunk a lot on Friday or Saturday night, but that did not make them alcoholics. Now, they do not have to go to work, and so they start drinking earlier and earlier in the day. Some people do this partly to drive away the symptoms of depression, but unfortunately, over time alcohol aggravates depression. Another reason people drink excessively after retirement is boredom. Depression and boredom are two real problems for many men who have not planned for retirement. Thus a history of the patient's use of alcohol is always important. Patients often deny drinking excessively, so relatives should be asked about indirect evidence such as empty bottles in the garbage can or bottles around the house.

Most of the other drugs a patient might be taking will be either prescribed or bought over the counter. Over-the-counter drugs frequently are not included in the drug history, because many elderly people do not consider such drugs medication. Yet the elderly are the largest single group of purchasers of such drugs, which include sleeping pills, laxatives, antihistamines, tonics, and antacids.

Many prescribed drugs cause confusion in the elderly. Particular offenders are psychoactive medications, (drugs that affect the mind), such as neuroleptic drugs, benzodiazepines, antidepressants, lithium, and hypnotic drugs. Such drugs have a prolonged action, especially in older patients because of the impaired functioning of the liver and kidneys. There also is evidence that the brain of the older individual is more sensitive to these drugs.

In a number of nursing homes many residents take a tranquilizer of one sort or another, although this often is more for the convenience of the staff than for any benefit to the resident. For example, many residents may have watched late-night television before entering the nursing home; however, institutional rules demand that residents retire at 9 PM. The medication is prescribed to ensure that the residents retire at this hour, as well as for other reasons. The ensuing sedation produces a state referred to as "mashed potato syndrome," so called because the resident is taking so many neuroleptic drugs that when lunch is served, she falls face first into her mashed potatoes.

In one case, a man was referred to a geriatric outreach program because two women had seen him standing naked on the balcony of an apartment building at 2 PM in midwinter. The women complained that he was a flasher. The social worker and physician who went to the apartment to investigate found an 80-year-old man in almost total darkness with all the shades drawn. His medicine cabinet revealed that he was taking amitriptyline (Elavil), imipramine (Tofranil), haloperidol (Haldol), thioridazine (Mellaril), promazine (Sparine, which by this time had been removed from the market), chlorpromazine (Thorazine), and diazepam (Valium).

The physician put all the drugs on the kitchen table and asked, "Now, Mr. Jones, which of these medications do you take?" Mr. Jones replied, "It depends on how I feel." The physician then asked, "Which ones did you take today?" The patient replied, "I took one of these, but I don't really remember, but I think I took two of the other ones, because they work really good and help me and I took one of the blue ones." The label on one of the bottles revealed that the prescription had been written by a doctor who had been dead for 5 years and who was dead when the medication was refilled. The prescription read, "Valium 5 mg q.i.d., ad lib," meaning the prescription could be refilled an unlimited number of times, even after the physician's death.

Mr. Jones had seen several physicians since his doctor had died, but he had never been asked what medication he was taking or what he had at home. No one ever instructed him to throw out the old medication; they just added a new one. This man's confusion was cured by discontinuing all his medication.

It is also important to remember that elderly patients borrow drugs from their neighbors. A 75-year-old man was seen in psychiatric consultation in the local hospital because of confusion that had come on in the previous 5 days. He was unable to answer questions, was confused, and delusional, and looked very ill. He was totally disoriented. Despite an intensive workup, which included a CT scan of the head, lumbar puncture, and EEG, no cause could be found for his delirium. The patient was thought to have Alzheimer's disease, and the psychiatric consultation was requested. While this consultation was taking place, a neighbor who knew the patient well entered the room and was asked what she thought had happened to him. She admitted that the patient had been borrowing pills from her "for swelling of the ankles." Because one pill didn't work, he had taken two and ended up taking three a day. The patient had borrowed a form of digitalis and was suffering from digitalis toxicity.

Many elderly people never throw old medications away because they've spent so much money on them. Consequently, as in the case of Mr. Jones, they may still be using medications prescribed months or years earlier, without informing the current physician. Elderly patients should be encouraged to show their physicians all the medications they are taking, including over-the-counter drugs, and physicians should be diligent in questioning patients about such medication.

"E" IS FOR EYES AND EARS

Some people appear confused because they cannot hear or see well. Out of self-consciousness they pretend they can hear, and they answer questions with something totally irrelevant, thus giving the impression of being demented. Also, some elderly people may be too vain to wear a hearing aid, and they may need to be confronted to be convinced of the need for one.

One such person was a psychiatrist in his eighties, and a close friend of the author. He did not want anyone to know he could not hear, yet whenever anyone had a conversation with him, particularly in a restaurant or other noisy place, he could not understand anything unless it was shouted. One day the author said to him, "Dan, everybody thinks you have Alzheimer's disease. You appear demented simply because you won't wear your hearing aid." From that time on, he wore the hearing aid.

The other special sense organ that is affected by aging is eyesight. When people start losing their vision, they may bump into things while walking across a room, making them appear to be confused. This problem is discussed further in Chapter 3.

"M" IS FOR METABOLIC AND ENDOCRINE DISEASE

Patients with uncontrolled diabetes mellitus and hypothyroidism often display confusional states. Diabetes mellitus can become uncontrolled for a number of reasons, including infection, dietary indiscretion, failure to take necessary medication, and use of sugar-containing medicines such as cough syrups.

Any imbalance in serum electrolytes may be manifested as impaired mental functions. Such an imbalance can be precipitated by a bout of diarrhea or by medications such as diuretic drugs, and lithium, a medication used in elderly patients with mood disorders that is notorious for producing delirium through electrolyte disturbance.

"E" IS FOR EMOTIONAL DISORDERS

Paranoid disorders and mood disorders are the two most common forms of psychiatric illness in the elderly that may be confused with Alzheimer's disease. Elderly individuals have a higher incidence of paranoid disorders than younger people.

Depression is common in the elderly. It is confused with Alzheimer's disease, because it does not manifest itself in the classical manner. Elderly patients who are depressed frequently have a list of somatic complaints, emotional withdrawal, or seeming confusion. The diagnosis of depression is made because of the abruptness of onset, the lack of animation in the patient, loss of appetite, and insomnia.

"N" IS FOR NUTRITIONAL DEFICIENCIES

Elderly people commonly do not eat wholesome meals and are likely to suffer from numerous nutritional deficiencies (dealt with further in Chapter 7). Patients with such deficiencies display confusion and other signs of dementia. Patients who have had bowel surgery are particularly at risk. It is sometimes difficult to obtain a history of such surgery, because the patient may have forgotten it and records may not be readily available. Some patients may be starving and suffering from ketosis.

"T" IS FOR TUMORS AND TRAUMA

Two of the biggest advances in the past 20 years were the CT scan and magnetic resonance imaging (MRI). Although these do not help much in the diagnosis of early Alzheimer's disease, they do help detect traumatic injury and tumors in the brain.

"I" IS FOR INFECTION

Elderly people often appear to be confused when they have an infection, and the picture may be further obscured if the individual does not have an elevated temperature. They may not be running a temperature. The two most common infections in the elderly that produce a dementia-like picture are pneumonia and urinary tract infections, which are discussed further in Chapter 3.

"A" IS FOR ARTERIOSCLEROSIS

Arteriosclerosis can lead to heart failure and insufficient blood supply to the heart or brain. The patient sometimes has bouts of confusion and heart failure and almost always experiences depression. As previously mentioned, these symptoms may masquerade as pseudodementia. Arteriosclerosis may also be responsible for strokes. If the stroke is large and affects the motor area of the brain, the patient has paralysis. Small strokes, on the other hand, may not be noticed until so many have occurred and sufficient brain tissue has been destroyed that a dementia results. This is called *multiinfarct dementia*, or MID. Unlike

Alzheimer's disease, it is abrupt in onset and progresses in a stepwise fashion rather than a steady decline.

MENTAL STATUS EXAMINATION

After the history, the next most important component of a patient evaluation is a mental status examination. The major purpose of this examination is to exclude other possible mental disorders.

Like the differential diagnosis, the mental status examination has a handy mnemonic: AMSIT. The "A" stands for appearance, general behavior and speech. The patient's appearance may point to impaired mental function. For example, a person who comes in wearing three pairs of pants, has most of the buttons on his shirt undone, has not knotted his tie, and has soup stains down the front of his suit is not likely to have normal mental functions.

Behavior may be easy to judge: Does the person sit still? Is he agitated? Does he keep moving around? Behavior toward the caregiver, as well as the examiner, during a combined interview is a useful indicator of brain function. Some patients are mute throughout the interview, yet appear to understand what is going on. Others may lash out at the caregiver or appear to have no interest whatsoever in the proceeding.

"M" stands for mood, with sadness or elation, the other end of the spectrum, of particular interest. Sometimes a person's relatives may believe he has Alzheimer's disease if he is very excited, talks rapidly, cannot seem to get his words out fast enough, and is elated. However, this is more likely to be a bipolar disorder than a dementia.

"S" stands for sensorium and refers to the person's orientation to time, place, and other people. A person loses sensorium in the reverse order in which it was learned. For example, the last thing a person learns is how to tell time, and this is the first thing that departs when the person begins to lose orientation. A child first learns to recognize parents and other significant people, then where she lives, and lastly how to tell time. These skills are lost in reverse order, so that disorientation to time is the first to manifest itself.

The "I" stands for intellectual functioning. The Mini Mental Status Examination* is a valuable tool in rapid evaluation of intellectual

---

* Cognitive capacity screening examination (Adapted from Jacobs, Bernhard, Delgado and Strain: Ann Int Med 86:40, 1977).

MINI-MENTAL STATUS EXAMINATION

Examiner _____ Date _____

Instructions: Check items answered correctly. Write incorrect or unusual answers in space provided. If necessary, urge patient once to complete task.

Introduction to patient: "I would like to ask you a few questions. Some you will find very easy and others may be very hard. Just do your best."

1. What day of the week is this? _____
2. What month? _____
3. What day of the month? _____
4. What year? _____
5. What place is this? _____
6. Repeat these numbers: 8, 7, 2. _____
7. Say them backwards. _____
8. Repeat these numbers: 6, 3, 7, 1. _____
9. Listen to these numbers: 6, 9, 4. Count 1 through 10 out loud, then repeat 6, 9, 4. (Help if needed. Then use numbers 5, 7, 3). _____
10. Listen to these numbers: 8, 1, 4, 3. Count 1 through 10 out loud, then repeat 8, 1, 4, 3. _____
11. Beginning with Sunday, say the days of the week backwards. _____
12. 9 + 3 is: _____
13. Add 6 (to the previous answer or "to 12"). _____
14. Take away 5 ("from 18"). Repeat these words after me and remember them. I will ask for them later: Hat, Car, Tree, Twenty-six. _____

15. The opposite of fast is slow. The opposite of up is: _____
16. The opposite of large is: _____
17. The opposite of hard is: _____
18. An orange and a banana are both fruits. Red and blue are both: _____
19. A penny and a dime are both: _____
20. What were those words I asked you to remember? (Hat) _____
21. (Car) _____
22. (Tree) _____
23. (Twenty-six) _____
24. Take away 7 from 100. Then take away 7 from what is left and keep going—100 − 7 is: _____
25. Minus 7 _____
26. Minus 7 (write down answers: check correct subtraction of 7) _____
27. Minus 7 _____
28. Minus 7 _____
29. Minus 7 _____
30. Minus 7 _____

TOTAL CORRECT (maximum score is 30). _____

Patient's occupation (previous, if not employed) _____

Education _____ Age _____

Circle estimated intelligence (based on education, occupation, and history, not on test score)

Below average   Average   Above average

Patient was: Cooperative _____
Uncooperative _____   Depressed _____
Lethargic _____   Other _____

Medical diagnosis: _____

Cognitive capacity screening examination (Adapted from Jacobs, et al.: Ann Int Med 86:40, 1977) functioning. It consists of 30 questions, some that test sensorium and others that test arithmetic, abstract thinking and memory. (The test is included in the box on p. 22.) With a literate patient with a high-school education, a score of less than 24 is highly suggestive of impaired intellectual functions. The test also indicates the severity of the disease.

The "T" stands for thinking processes. Patients with Alzheimer's disease demonstrate changes in almost all of the categories included under this section. Early in the disease most patients have difficulty focusing on a goal and often are circumstantial or tangential in their thinking; that is, when asked questions, they tend to give answers that may contain a lot of extraneous details but that do not directly answer the question. Later in the course of the disease much of a patient's thinking is illogical or incoherent or both.

As a rule, delusions and hallucinations do not occur until the disease is fairly advanced. The hallucinations frequently are visual and sometimes frightening, such as seeing smoke or flames when none exist. The delusions often are of strangers being in the house or of people from the past coming to visit, and they occur because the patient does not recognize familiar objects or people. Abstracting ability almost always is affected fairly early in the disease. The patient with Alzheimer's disease gives concrete responses when asked proverbs or when asked to state what is familiar about common objects. Social judgment frequently is impaired, and insight is almost always absent.

LABORATORY TESTS

A diagnostic accuracy of about 80% can be achieved on the purely clinical portions of the examinations; the addition of laboratory tests increases this rate to about 90%. The following tests are recommended (and described in the glossary):
CT scan of the brain
Chest x-ray film
Comprehensive biochemical screening (autoanalysis of the blood)
Blood count and vitamin B_{12} level
Thyroid function tests
Electrocardiogram (ECG)
Human immunodeficiency virus (AIDS) test
Additional tests that may be useful in some instances include the following:
EEG
Lumbar puncture

MRI of the brain

Positron emission tomography (PET) scan of the brain

Occasionally a patient must be referred for psychological testing. Neuropsychologists particularly can be helpful in differentiating between Alzheimer's disease and other brain disorders that cannot be distinguished either by laboratory tests or the usual clinical measures. A group of tests known as the Halstead-Reitan Battery is especially helpful in making such distinctions. Tests of this type are discussed further in Chapter 24.

In summary, the diagnosis of Alzheimer's disease currently is in a state of flux. The diagnosis traditionally has been made on clinical grounds with supporting laboratory data. However, some of the new techniques such as positron emission tomography and magnetic resonance imaging, which are available only in large centers, may prove valuable in the future. It is also likely that a specific protein is involved in Alzheimer's disease and that it is present in the cerebrospinal fluid. In the near future it may be possible to assay this abnormal proteins routinely.

BIBLIOGRAPHY

American Psychiatric Association: Diagnostic and statistical manual of mental disorders, ed III-R, Washington, DC, The Association.

Drayer BP: Imaging of the aging brain. I. Normal findings. II. Pathological conditions, Radiology 166(3):785-796, 797-806, 1988.

Erkinjuntti T et al: Dementia among medical inpatients, Arch Intern Med 146:1923-1926, 1986.

Folstein MF and Whitehouse PJ: Cognitive impariment of Alzheimer disease, Neurobehav Toxicol Teratol 5(6):631-634, 1983.

Friedland R et al: The diagnosis of Alzheimer-type dementia, JAMA 252(19):2750-2752, 1984.

Kerzner LJ: Diagnosis and treatment of Alzheimer's disease, Adv Intern Med 29:447-470, 1984.

Larson EB et al: Diagnostic evaluation of 200 elderly outpatients with suspected dementia, J Gerontol 40(5): 536-543, 1985.

McKhann G et al: Clinical diagnosis of Alzheimer's disease: report of the NINCDS-ADRDA Work Group, Neurology 34:939-944, 1984.

Spinnler H and Della Sala S: The role of clinical neuropsychology in the neurological diagnosis of Alzheimer's disease, J Neurol 235(5):258-271, 1988.

Toseland RW, Derico A, and Owen ML: Alzheimer's disease and related disorders: assessment and intervention, Health Soc Work 9(3):212-226, 1984.

3

Factors that aggravate Alzheimer's disease

R. Hamdy

Currently Alzheimer's disease is believed to be an irreversible, slowly progressive process characterized by gradual deterioration. Nevertheless, not infrequently a patient who is known to have Alzheimer's disease will deteriorate suddenly. The patient's relatives and even some physicians and nurses may attribute this sudden downturn to the underlying Alzheimer's disease process, but this often is not the case. In many instances some other specific disease is responsible for the rapid deterioration.

It is important to detect any factor that may worsen the patient's mental and/or physical state, since many of these factors are reversible if treated early. If not detected in time, they may lead to further irreversible deterioration.

A person's mental functions are controlled by the brain, which is made up of a number of nerve cells, or neurons. Brain functioning depends on the number of brain cells and their integrity and on the efficiency of the blood circulation. Since neurons have no nutrition stores, they depend entirely on the circulation to provide them with adequate quantities of glucose, oxygen, and various other nutrients. Similarly, an efficient circulation removes from the brain any waste or toxic substances that have been formed by the brain cells through their metabolic activity.

Thus if the blood circulation is ineffective, not only will the nerve cells be deprived of various nutrients, but also various waste or toxic substances will accumulate in or around the nerve cells. The nerve cells cannot function properly under these conditions, and the patient's mental impairment may worsen. For instance, the patient may become confused, lethargic, apathetic, and drowsy, or he may become irritable, violent, and aggressive. Since patients with Alzheimer's disease already have a reduced number of brain cells, they are particularly vulnerable to a number of factors that may interfere with the functions of the remaining nerve cells. In healthy older individuals these factors may not lead to any deterioration of the mental functions, but they may be of sufficient magnitude to affect patients with Alzheimer's disease. These factors include the following:

1. Sudden reduction in the number of neurons
2. Sudden decrease in the blood supply to the brain
3. Diminished quality of blood reaching the brain
4. Altered sensory perceptions
5. Drugs
6. Other influences

SUDDEN REDUCTION IN THE NUMBER OF NEURONS

To function properly, the brain must have a minimum number of healthy cells. In Alzheimer's disease, brain cells progressively die. If in addition the number of neurons is suddenly reduced, the patient's mental state may deteriorate abruptly. A number of conditions may be responsible for this loss of neurons, including strokes, subdural hematomas, and space-occupying lesions in the skull.

Strokes (Cerebrovascular Accidents)

When a patient suffers a stroke, the blood supply to part of the brain is suddenly interrupted and the brain cells in that part die. Strokes have three main causes for:

- A thrombus, or blood clot, which forms inside the blood vessel and usually complicates abnormalities in the blood vessels themselves, such as arteriosclerosis or a stenotic (narrowed) lesion.
- An embolus, which is part of a blood clot that becomes detached and circulates with the blood stream until it becomes impacted in one of the small arteries
- A hemorrhage, which occurs when a blood vessel ruptures. In this instance, not only is the blood flow to that part of the brain interrupted, but also blood accumulates in the brain, compressing and destroying neighboring brain cells.

In about two thirds of patients over 65 years of age who suffer strokes, the cause of the stroke is a thrombus; in the other one third, the stroke is the result of an embolus. Cerebral hemorrhages are rare in old age.

The signs of a stroke depend on which part of the brain is affected. Large strokes, particularly those affecting the motor functions, have a dramatic presentation, with the patient developing speech difficulties or the paralysis of the arm or leg. Smaller strokes may not give rise to paralysis and may go unnoticed. They also may interfere only marginally with a patient's mental functions until so many have developed and so much brain tissue has been destroyed that the patient's mental functions become severely impaired; this is the underlying process of multiinfarct dementia. Although currently little can be done once a stroke occurs, a number of therapeutic measures can be taken to prevent additional strokes.

Subdural Hematomas

A subdural hematoma is a hemorrhage inside the skull but outside the brain. Characteristically, subdural hematomas complicate head injuries. In most instances the trauma itself is relatively minor, such as a fall in the bathtub. The manifestations often are not obvious until a few days or even weeks later, and by then the patient or caregivers may have forgotten all about it. Even if the trauma is severe enough to render the patient unconscious, he usually recovers consciousness and may appear normal for a few days or weeks, before subtle changes develop. In contrast, patients with Alzheimer's disease may have a much more dramatic presentation. Immediately after the injury, the patient may not appear any worse than usual, but a few days or weeks later symptoms usually are severe and may include a significant change in personality, apathy, lethargy, irritability, aggressiveness, and even violence.

The time gap between trauma and impairment of mental functions occurs because the initial hemorrhage is limited in size or because the bleeding stops. With time, however, the hemorrhage turns into a blood clot, which starts drawing fluid from the surrounding tissues (by osmosis) and grows larger. As this happens, pressure is exerted on the brain tissue and symptoms develop.

Space-Occupying Lesions in the Skull

Unlike most other cavities in the body, the skull (the cranial cavity) has a constant volume that is mostly occupied by the brain. If a patient develops a brain abscess or metastases (secondary cancer growths) in the brain, these "space occupying lesions" can grow only at the expense of the brain, which at first becomes compressed and later may be destroyed. Patients with Alzheimer's disease, who already have a reduced number of brain cells, are particularly vulnerable to space-occupying lesions in the skull.

SUDDEN DECREASE IN THE BLOOD SUPPLY TO THE BRAIN

As previously mentioned, the brain depends completely on the blood circulation for the oxygen, glucose, and other nutrients it needs. Even though enough neurons may be present for the brain to function at a certain level, mental functions can deteriorate as the cerebral (brain) blood flow is reduced. Interestingly, although the brain represents only about 2% of the body weight, it receives about 15% of the quantity of blood pumped by the heart and uses about 25% of the total inhaled oxygen.

Circulation of blood through the body is maintained by the heart. The quantity of blood pumped by the heart in 1 minute is known as the cardiac output. A number of conditions can reduce the cardiac output, including myocardial infarctions and arrythmias.

Myocardial Infarctions

In myocardial infarction part of the heart muscle is deprived of its blood supply. As a result, this part of the heart muscle dies. If the area destroyed is large enough, the overall function of the heart may be disrupted and the amount of blood pumped during each contraction will be reduced. The effect of this reduction may be magnified if the heart rate is changed. (See next section, "Arrythmias.") As a result, the heart will not be able to maintain an adequate cardiac output, leading to a decrease in the amount of blood reaching various parts of the body, including the brain. Should this condition arise in a patient with Alzheimer's disease whose brain functions are already jeopardized, the patient's mental functions are likely to deteriorate considerably.

In contrast to the classical picture that develops in younger people, the elderly may suffer a myocardial infarction without having any chest pain. This sometimes is called a "silent myocardial infarction." In the elderly the only sign of myocardial infarction may be a bout of confusion or dizziness or a fall.

Arrhythmias (Irregular Heart Rate)

At rest the heart of an older person beats about 65 times a minute, a little faster than one beat per second. The heart actually functions in cycles, each cycle consisting of a contraction (systole), during which the blood in the heart is forcefully ejected into the arteries, and a period of relaxation (diastole), during which blood returns to the heart through the veins. Whereas systole is an active process, diastole is mostly a passive one, allowing the heart muscles to relax and get ready for the next contraction. In normal, healthy people, the amount of blood ejected during systole is the same as that received by the heart during diastole.

When the heart rate increases, both the systolic and diastolic periods are relatively shortened. At high rates, however, the diastolic period tends to be shortened more than the systolic period. This interferes with the amount of blood that fills the heart during diastole and in turn reduces the amount of blood pumped when the heart contracts. In an attempt to maintain a constant cardiac output, the heart beats even faster. At these very high rates, the cardiac output cannot be maintained and may actually fall because of the markedly reduced diastolic period. Elderly people are much more vulnerable than younger people to the effects of a change in heart rhythm (arrhythmia).

DIMINISHED QUALITY OF BLOOD REACHING THE BRAIN

Since the brain depends entirely on the blood for the oxygen and nutrients it needs to function properly, it is easy to see that, even if the number of brain cells is adequate and the blood flow (circulation) is effective, mental functions may become impaired if the quality of the blood reaching the brain is not adequate. Because patients with Alzheimer's disease already have a reduced number of brain cells, they are particularly vulnerable to any such change, which may be caused by reduced oxygenation of the blood, reduced blood glucose, or toxic compounds in the bloodstream.

Reduced Oxygenation of the Blood

As the blood passes through the lungs, the hemoglobin molecules in the red blood corpuscles take up oxygen. The oxygenated blood returns to the heart, which pumps it to other parts of the body, including the brain. If the blood is not oxygenated adequately in the lungs, less oxygen will be carried to the rest of the body, meaning that less will reach the brain.

Blood oxygenation in the lungs can be inadequate for a number of reasons, including respiratory tract infections (pneumonias); pulmonary embolisms (small pieces of blood clots in the lungs); chronic obstructive airway diseases (asthma and emphysema); pulmonary neoplasia (cancer of the lungs); pleural effusions (accumulation of fluid between the lungs and the chest wall); and pneumothorax (accumulation of air between the lungs and the chest wall).

Anemia also can reduce the amount of oxygen circulating with the blood. In anemia the number of red blood cells and the total quantity of circulating hemoglobin are reduced; therefore, the amount of oxygen that can be carried by the blood also is reduced.

Reduced Blood Glucose (Hypoglycemia)

Since brain cells have no glucose stores, a sudden reduction in the blood glucose level would leave them unable to function properly, resulting in impaired mental functions. Hypoglycemia mainly occurs when a patient receives an overdose of insulin or when he receives a normal dose but skips a meal. Less frequently, orally administered hypoglycemic agents used to control diabetes mellitus may induce hypoglycemia.

Toxic Substances in the Bloodstream

Even during normal functioning, the body produces a number of potentially toxic substances that are either changed to less toxic compounds or are eliminated from the body. If the organs that transform or eliminate these substances (primarily the kidneys and the liver) are impaired, the toxic compounds accumulate.

Impaired renal functions

One of the kidney's main functions is to rid the body of many toxic substances, especially the water-soluble ones, by excreting them in the urine. As mentioned previously, if the kidneys do not work properly, these toxic substances accumulate. A number of factors can cause renal impairment, including the following:

Drugs, particularly antihypertensive agents, nonsteroidal antiinflammatory agents, analgesics, and antibiotics

Dehydration, a not uncommon condition, especially in older patients whose sense of thirst often appears to be blunted

Infections

Impaired hepatic function

Whereas the kidneys eliminate water-soluble compounds by excreting them in the urine, the liver eliminates water insoluble or fat-soluble toxic compounds by excreting them with bile or by conjugating them with compounds that make them water soluble, to be excreted at a later stage by the kidneys. Alcohol abuse is one of the main causes of impaired hepatic function. Hepatic impairment also may be caused by certain drugs, especially those metabolized (broken down) in the liver, such as most tranquilizers, sedatives, and other compounds that act on the central nervous system.

Infection

If a patient develops an infection, regardless of its location, toxic compounds are likely to accumulate in the body, circulate with the bloodstream, and reach the brain, possibly interfering with the brain's functioning. This may produce an acute confusional state in the patient. If the infection is in the chest, not only do toxic products accumulate, but also the amount of oxygen in the blood often is diminished, since the lung congestion that complicates such infections interferes with the free passage of oxygen molecules. Chest infections are notorious for giving rise to confusional states in elderly people. Although individuals who do not have Alzheimer's disease sometimes become confused as a result of chest infections, the confusion tends to be much more severe in patients with the disease.

It is important to know that chest infections frequently are difficult to diagnose in older people, because most of the characteristic symptoms and signs seen in younger adults are absent. Such signs include fever, tachycardia (rapid heart rate), and cough with expectoration of sputum, as well as the characteristic findings detected during the clinical examination and on the x-ray films.

An older person with a chest infection may not have a fever; often the temperature-regulating center in the brain does not function properly in old age and is less sensitive than in youth. This may be one reason why elderly people are more likely to develop hypothermia. Similarly, an increased heart rate may not be observed if some disorder in the heart's conduction tissue prevents it from increasing its rate. Cough and expectoration of sputum may be absent if the patient is dehydrated. Alternatively, cough and expectoration of sputum may have been present for some time if the patient has a chronic obstructive airway disease. Similarly, the characteristic physical findings may be obscured by dehydration, kyphosis, and kyphoscoliosis.

The latter two conditions may also mask the characteristic radiological features.

One of the most important signs in the diagnosis of chest infections in old age is an increased respiratory rate. Unfortunately, this sign is often overlooked and when counted is often approximated. A rapid respiratory rate may be the only sign of a chest infection in an older person. It is ironic that this single sign usually is the one that is given the least importance during the clinical examination and subsequent observation of the patient.

Subacute bacterial endocarditis (SBE) is another cause of confusion and impaired mental functioning in old age, specially in patients with Alzheimer's disease. In SBE the heart valves are infected, and the heart may be unable to maintain an adequate circulation. In addition, bacteria and their toxic products circulate with the blood (bacteremia and toxemia) and further interfere with the patient's mental functions. SBE is insidious in onset and progresses slowly. The diagnosis usually is not made until fairly late, when the disease is well established.

ALTERED MESSAGES FROM THE ENVIRONMENT

To react appropriately in any situation, a person must be able to perceive and understand a number of messages received from the environment. For example, a normal person who wakes up at 2 AM will not set about preparing breakfast for the whole household; even if he does not know what time it was, he will check a clock, realize the time, and try to go back to sleep. Even if no clock were available, he might guess that it is too early to get out of bed, let alone fix breakfast. If, on the other hand, his vision is poor, he may not be able to read the time on the clock accurately and may think it is time to get up. A person's preceptions can be altered by impaired vision and hearing, a sudden change in surroundings, and pain and discomfort.

Impaired Vision

In most instances vision is the prime factor that determines a person's behavior. For example, if a person notices black particles in his food while eating, his immediate reaction depends on what he thinks the particles are. This is mostly governed by his visual acuity and his ability to correlate what is actually seen with past visual experiences. Similarly, a person's reaction to someone who knocks on the door and identifies himself as a sales representative will largely be governed by the customer's perception of the salesman and whether he "looks honest." On a more basic level, simply finding the way to the restroom, for example, depends largely on visual acuity.

If the light rays that enter the eyes are abnormally distorted, as may happen with cataracts and glaucoma, the patient's perception of objects may be erroneous, and this may lead him to see things that are not really there; that is, to have illusions. This is particularly likely to happen if the patient is not fully conscious, as may occur if he has received sedative or hypnotic preparations or if he awakens in the middle of the night or is confused for any other reason. Visual impairment is discussed further in Chapter 22.

Impaired Hearing

Any deterioration in a patient's hearing may interfere with conversational ability: the patient may misinterpret questions and give inappropriate answers. Furthermore, if the patient experiences buzzing in his ears (because of wax or other diseases), he may be under the impression that someone is talking to him. If, his eyesight is also poor, he may think that a shadow is a person talking to him. Impaired auditory acuity is also discussed further in Chapter 22.

As an individual ages, visual and auditory acuity gradually deteriorates. If the patient also has a sudden deterioration in eyesight or hearing, he may become or appear to have become confused or disoriented and to have impaired mental functions. The individual thus may not be able to perceive his environment accurately and may make errors of judgment.

Sudden Change In Surroundings

A sudden change in surroundings often is confusing to older people, especially those suffering from Alzheimer's disease. This frequently is the case when a patient is first admitted to a nursing home or other, similar institution, where the patient may not recognize any of his surroundings. This is particularly likely to happen when a patient wakes up at night and finds himself in a strange environment. During the day he may recognize his environment, but in the dark after just awakening, he may not remember right away that he is in a new situation. This confusion may also happen when a patient with Alzheimer's disease is taken away from his familiar environment to spend a few days with a relative.

Pain and Discomfort

In a patient who is confused, pain and discomfort may significantly increase the degree of confusion and may impair the patient's mental functions. This is particularly the case when the patient is unable to understand or describe his pain or discomfort.

Common causes of discomfort include a full bladder, urinary incontinence, a full rectum, constipation, fecal incontinence and decubiti. Hunger and thirst also are uncomfortable sensations, as are being too hot or too cold or lying on crumpled sheets or foreign objects such as food debris. Pain is caused by a number of diseases, including osteoarthritis, leg cramps, and infections.

DRUGS

Not infrequently, prescribed medications can aggravate mental impairment. Drugs that act on the central nervous system such as hypnotics, sedatives, and tranquillizers, are particular offenders. There is considerable evidence that older people are much more susceptible to these drugs than younger patients, largely because an older person's body cannot get rid of the drug as quickly, either through excretion by the kidneys or break down by the liver. Thus it is important whenever these drugs are prescribed that they be given in the smallest effective dose. If necessary, the dosage can be adjusted according to the patient's response. Also, short-duration drugs are preferrable, since older patients tend to metabolize and excrete drugs more slowly.

Many over-the-counter drugs contain compounds that can sedate a patient. Besides sleeping preparations such drugs include many cold remedies, antiallergic medications, and even some antacids and anti-diarrhetic mixtures. If these drugs are given to the patient in large doses or in conjunction with other medications, drug overdose may result, and the patient's confusional state may worsen.

It must also be remembered that alcohol is a potent sedative and that it often potentiates the action of many other drugs. Drinking an excessive amount of alcohol may cause discomfort by increasing the volume of urine produced, thereby distending the bladder, and by precipitating dehydration.

Many other drugs may interfere with a patient's mental activities; for example, by altering the blood electrolytes (diuretics), precipitating anemia (drugs that irritate the gastrointestinal mucosa), inducing heart failure, precipitating cardiac irregularities, and reducing the blood pressure or the blood glucose level.

Because drug-induced confusion and impaired mental function are so common in old age, it is paramount that the physician be aware of all medications the patient is taking, whether prescribed, bought over the counter, or borrowed from others.

OTHER INFLUENCES
Physical Restraints

Physical restraints are often used to control abnormal behavior and to prevent the patient from injuring himself. Although restraints are necessary for a very small number of patients, they generally are overused. Injudicious use of restraints aggravates a patient's irritability, frustration, and confusion.

Sleep Deprivation

Sleep deprivation is a known and common cause of confusion, not only in older patients with Alzheimer's disease, but in any age group. This is further discussed in Chapter 4.

Other Medical Conditions

A number of diseases may cause a confusional state particularly in elderly people Some of these diseases were described earlier in this chapter; others were dealt with in Chapter 2. It is important to ensure that no medical condition is responsible for a patient's deteriorating mental state before assuming that the deterioration is secondary to Alzheimer's disease.

Because patients with Alzheimer's disease can suffer from a number of other diseases that may considerably worsen their mental and physical impairment, caregivers must be aware of this fact and report any sudden deterioration to the physician, who will try to identify the cause. Often the cause is reversible, and the patient's condition may improve once the disorder has been identified and treated. Alzheimer's disease progresses slowly and insidiously and seldom is the cause of sudden deterioration in a patient's condition.

BIBLIOGRAPHY

Moran MG and Thompson TL II: Changes in the aging brain as they affect psychotropics: a review, Int J Psychiatry Med 19(2):137-144, 1988.
Scott RB and Mitchell MC: Aging, alcohol, and the liver, J Am Geriatr Soc 36(3):255-265, 1988.

Straatsma BR et al: Aging-related cataract: laboratory investigation and clinical management, Ann Intern Med 102(1):82-92, 1985.

Tyers AG: Aging and the ocular adnexa: a review, J R Soc Med 75(11):900-902, 1982.

Veith RC and Raskind MA: The neurobiology of aging: does it predispose to depression? Neurobiol Aging 9(1):101-117, 1988.

Walsh DA: Aging and visual information processing: potential implications for everyday seeing. Part I. J Am Optom Assoc 59(4):301-306, 1988.

4

Special issues in the management of Alzheimer's disease

J. Turnbull and W. Wood

A key factor that caregivers must keep in mind when working with a patient with Alzheimer's disease (or any other dementing illness) is the patient's changing degree of adaptability, since adaptability gradually declines as the illness progresses. Changing adaptability is a key concept. The continuum of deteriorating function in Alzheimer's disease often is compared to its opposite, the development of coping skills in childhood. There is a period in a person's life when he reaches the peak of adaptability; from that point begins a decline that is hastened by physical or mental dysfunction, and very often both are present in the patient with Alzheimer's disease.

Many of the factors that are important in the management of patients with dementia involve preserving a stable environment. Patients with dementia have a progressive sensitivity to any changes in environment, physical function, and mental function, and such changes often are reflected in behavioral changes. One leading factor that may be reflected in behavioral change is the use of medication that may benefit a particular physical problem but that may adversely affect behavior and cognitive function. Another factor comprises the problems created for patients and caregivers by disturbances in sleep and the sleep/wake cycle. These issues are considered later in this chapter.

MANIPULATING THE ENVIRONMENT

In evaluating the environment for factors that might be changed to improve the patient's condition, the caregiver must keep in mind the patient's stage in the Alzheimer's disease process. With the onset of the dementing illness, it is important to stabilize the environment, to provide comfort, and to reduce the amount of frustration that the individual may face in daily life.

A patient's environment may be stabilized by having him attend to the activities of daily life according to a set routine. Regular hours should be established for eating, sleeping, bathing, going out, and receiving visitors. In the late stages of the disease, patients may require absolutely no changes in the immediate environment. Overnight trips or even changing a patient's room may produce confusion so severe that it takes days to correct. When the patient is getting dressed, limiting the number of choices is very helpful, such as allowing him to pick only one or two articles.

It is also important to provide the patient with increasing stimulation, and as the disease progresses the task becomes harder and harder. This stimulation must be provided even if the patient rejects it or if it is not acknowledged by any response. Some caregivers have found that simply getting the patient's attention, getting him to look them in the face, for example, requires more and more effort. The situation moves from simply speaking to the patient and having him turn to look at the speaker, to having to put a hand on his shoulder or move around in front of him. If the patient is looking down, the caregiver may have to bend down and confront him, looking him directly in the face, to make contact. Otherwise the patient tends to ignore the speaker, a frustrating act often perceived as willful and deliberate. Stimulation for the patient with Alzheimer's disease has been systematized into a program called "reality orientation," which is discussed in Chapter 20.

Initially the patient with Alzheimer's disease may be able to shower and shave but may dress inappropriately, or he may be able to shower and dress but may forget to shave. It may take many reminders for the patient to finish getting ready to go out, and soon he becomes frustrated. The caregiver also may become exasperated and tend to treat the patient like a child using such unhelpful cajoling as, "I told you to. . . ." It would be more helpful for the caregiver to accompany the patient to the bathroom and say, "OK, this is what we need to do now." The frustration on both sides stems from unreasonable expectations of what the patient can accomplish.

As the disease progresses, the patient begins to have difficulty choosing clothing and accomplishing relatively minor tasks that require sequential reasoning. Memory is significantly impaired, and socialization declines. The patient's response to the environment is diminished, and he may simply sit in a chair for hours on end. A person who might have been very active, taking afternoon walks, getting out and working in the yard, and doing all sorts of things that took up a great deal of time may be unable or unwilling to pursue these activities. At this point the individual needs more attention, even though he is responding less to such attention.

The patient's seeming lack of appreciation for the caretaker's efforts may also pose problems. An important principle in motivating human interaction is appreciation, as reflected by a smile, a nod, or a change in expression. A patient in stage 3 of Alzheimer's disease may show no such response and may have a totally blank, expressionless face. He may not make eye contact with the caregiver after she has worked very hard to fix a special meal or has taken time out from her activities to do something extra for the patient. This situation requires a great deal of understanding on the part of the caregiver, something that can be very difficult in an institution, where a caregiver may look after many patients who are unable to say "thank you," as other people would.

As the disease progresses, the patient needs more and more physical care. He may be unable to bathe and very often must be treated like a small child in all his basic daily functions. Caretakers with small children may be struck by the similarities in caring for these children and the adult. Individuals who must care both for children and for elderly people with dementia have sometimes been called "the sandwich generation."

Sleep

Unfortunately, many elderly people have trouble getting to sleep. In fact, many clinicians report that insomnia is a complaint of more than half the population aged 65 or older. Twice as many people over 65 years of age use hypnotic drugs regularly as do those 30 to 55 years of age. Far from solving the problem, these drugs frequently cause unwanted side effects, which are even more likely to be serious if the elderly person has Alzheimer's disease.

Normal sleep

Sleep is a state consisting of two alternating and distinct substates, each of which occurs several times a night. Non-rapid eye movement sleep (NREM), which is further divided into stages one through four, occurs about 75% of the night of sleep. Rapid eye movement sleep (REM), during which most dreams take place, accounts for the remaining 25%. As a person ages, the duration of these sleep stages changes. Less total time is spent in actual sleep and less time in REM sleep. However, the elderly individual also tends to spend more time in bed than his 35-year-old counterpart.

The most common sleep complaints in the elderly are an inability to stay asleep and early arousal. In young adults, in contrast, lying awake a long time and trying to get to sleep are more common. Sleep problems in an elderly person are compounded by social isolation, boredom, physical illness, and sensory deprivation.

CASE EXAMPLE

One of our fathers, who is 84-years old, is in excellent physical and mental health except for a moderate hearing loss. When he comes to visit me in Tennessee from his home in Vancouver, British Columbia, he always remarks, "I seem to sleep so much better here in Tennessee. Do you suppose it's the air?"

At his home in Vancouver, isolated much of the time, increasingly hard of hearing and, during the winter (when he cannot garden his allotment), bored, he tends to look to sleep to ease the cares of the day. The frequent awakenings and poor sleep maintenance are seen as problems, but when visiting his family they are minor inconveniences because his days are filled with activity and socialization.

Evaluating insomnia

Sleep is often ignored during the medical or nursing inquiry. In the patient with Alzheimer's disease, the information must be obtained from relatives or caretakers who live with the patient. It should include the following:

Number of hours spent trying to sleep
Number of daytime naps
Number of hours of sleep desired
Medications taken regularly (prescribed and over the counter)
Time taken to fall asleep
Number of nocturnal awakenings

Because most individuals are poor sleep historians, the patient or his relatives should be encouraged to keep a sleep journal. This will serve as an accurate record of sleeping habits that can be assessed and analyzed. Through sleep histories physicians can distinguish difficulty falling asleep (DFA), multiple awakenings, early morning awakenings (EMAs), and day-night reversal.

DFA is often caused by anxiety, ruminating, and obsessive worrying. It is a characteristic of early Alzheimer's disease when the individual recognizes his increasing difficulty with failing memory. Multiple awakenings and early morning awakenings are more characteristic of depression, although they, too, may occur early in Alzheimer's disease. It is not uncommon for depression and the dementia of early Alzheimer's disease to occur concurrently.

Etiology of insomnia. The causes of insomnia can generally be divided into four groups:

1. Biological predisposition
2. Drugs
3. Disturbing environment
4. Bad habits

The sleep difficulty may be caused by a painful problem such as arthritis, angina, or a gastrointestinal ailment. Other medical conditions such as asthma, sleep apnea, irregular heart rate, and kidney or bladder disease also may cause insomnia.

A variety of drugs interfere with sleep. Among those that have been implicated are over-the-counter preparations with caffeine, alcohol, thyroid preparations, estrogen and progesterone preparations such as conjugate estrogen (Premarin) and Medroxyprogesterone acetate (Provera), and stimulant antidepressants such as methylphenidate (Ritalin) and fluoxetine (Prozac).

One commonly overlooked drug that causes insomnia in the elderly is caffeine. It is present not only in coffee and tea but also in many soft drinks, including Coca Cola, Pepsi Cola, and Fanta Orange.

Patients with Alzheimer's disease often have poor sleep habits. Some may exercise too close to the hour of sleep or may eat rich foods at bedtime. Others may have problems with noise or light coming in the window or with poor temperature control. Some individuals' homes are simply unsafe, and they may lie awake worrying that the house or apartment may be broken into.

Poor sleep habits also arise in patients with Alzheimer's disease who suffer from day-night reversal and get up at night. This is particularly perplexing and disturbing to relatives.

After carefully taking a history that considers the conditions mentioned, the physician often is left with nothing to treat but the symptoms themselves. In the elderly it is important to try to avoid hypnotic agents, which are simply too toxic for most elderly people. They accumulate in the body and cause daytime drowsiness and unsteadiness.

CASE EXAMPLE

A 69-year-old woman took 30 mg of flurazepam (Dalmane) every night for 7 weeks. One morning, while putting on her makeup, she fell and struck her chin on the sink, fracturing her jaw and knocking out four teeth. The only reason for her collapse was the Dalmane she had been taking. She had noticed some unsteadiness for several days previously and her speech was also beginning to slur. She had no further difficulties when her medication was discontinued.

Recommendations

It is important to remember that the elderly always sleep less well than they did when they were younger; this must be explained to them and to their relatives. Sleeping pills are not the answer for insomnia.

The following steps are recommended for helping an elderly patient achieve a good night's sleep:

1. Elderly individuals should not be allowed to oversleep and then attempt to catch up. Oversleeping resets the biological time clock and aggravates insomnia.
2. If an elderly person awakens prematurely, the caregiver should tell him to relax and try to let sleep return. In the early stages of Alzheimer's disease, patients may be encouraged to get up and read, watch television, or listen to a radio turned to low volume. The patient should return to bed if he feels sleepy. In late stages of the disease, patients should be stimulated to stay awake during the day and should be put to bed as late as possible.
3. Alcohol, smoking, and caffeine should be avoided in the afternoon or early evening before going to bed.
4. If the patient is a worrywart, the caregiver should get him to spend some time worrying in the early evening. We ask some of our patients to set aside 1 hour each day for worrying. The caregiver could say, for example, "I really want you to worry about your kids, your grandchildren, the bills, and all what ifs you can cram into 1 hour!"
5. The elderly person should experiment in the bedroom with lighting, low music, air conditioning, heating, heavier drapes, and so forth to discover what is comfortable for him.
6. A heavy meal should not be eaten within 2 hours of bedtime.
7. Regular exercise is vital for the patient with Alzheimer's disease, but it should not be scheduled too close to bedtime.
8. The patient should not nap during the day.
9. Caregivers can teach relaxation techniques even to patients with early stages of Alzheimer's disease.
10. If none of the common techniques seem to work, the patient

might seek help from a sleep disorders clinic. The nearest clinic can be obtained by writing to the Association of Sleep Disorders Centers, National Office, 604 Second Street, N.W., Rochester, MN 55902.

MANAGING THE IRRITABLE, AGGRESSIVE, OR VIOLENT PATIENT

There is no single approach to managing a patient who is violent or aggressive. However, a number of steps are useful.

The first step is a careful assessment of the patient in the environment. This step is sometimes overlooked by caregivers who react to the "aberrant" behavior without trying to discover why it occurred and who thus become prejudiced toward the aggressive patient for fear of being hurt themselves. In assessing a patient who is being aggressive toward caregivers or other patients, the first question to be addressed is what event precipitated the behavior. Sometimes it is difficult to explain the behavior. For example, undressing a patient for a bath may spark a violent outburst or aggressive resistance. This is not hard to understand in a patient late in the course of the disease; most people probably would react violently if a stranger walked up and started to unbutton their shirt and pants.

Aggressive behavior is a normal response in people who perceive that they are being threatened, and this is precisely what patients with Alzheimer's may be doing: defending themselves against a perceived threat.

Caregivers may prevent an aggressive reaction by taking a few minutes to introduce themselves to the patient and to explain what they are doing and what the patient can expect to happen next. No matter what the cause of the delirium, dementia, psychosis, or drug toxity, the caregiver's approach should be the same: Initiate action slowly, and make no sudden movements.

A second question in assessing aggressive or violent behavior is whether the patient behaves this way toward everyone or just toward specific individuals. For example, a patient who had served in the Korean War became aggressive toward Oriental nurses, believing, in his confused state, that they were "the enemy." Simply using other nurses when he required care alleviated this particular problem.

In some cases old childhood fears may be exacerbated because the patient misperceives common objects, which take on a threatening quality. A sock on the floor may be seen as a snake, or increasing darkness may be equated with going blind or going to sleep and never waking up.

Sometimes the explanation for aggressive behavior lies in the patient rather than the environment. Pain or discomfort, which may not be complained of directly, causes aggressive behavior if the patient feels that nothing is being done to help him. Patients with Alzheimer's disease also may not understand why they are hurting or what is causing the pain, and they may behave like a child by simply crying out or striking out. This pain may be caused by something as simple as a full bladder, an object sticking into the skin, a muscle cramp, or a joint that has stiffened through immobility.

Not infrequently, aggressive behavior also results from a delirium superimposed upon the dementia of Alzheimer's disease. This delirium may stem from any of the causes described in Chapter 2, such as a febrile illness, drugs, or metabolic disorders. When present, it exacerbates the patient's usual confusion and makes his world less tolerable and more threatening.

When all else fails, the management approaches that remain are medication, behavior modification, and, as a last resort, some form of restraint. When used, medication is generally of the sedating type. Both neuroleptic drugs and benzodiazepines have their place. However, medication is overused in most instances and is not without hazard. The neuroleptic drug most often prescribed for the aggressive or violent patient with Alzheimer's disease is haloperidol (Haldol). It must be used with care, since not only does it cause sedation, it also is very anticholinergic, causing dry mouth, blurred vision, urinary retention, and constipation. In general, "start low and go slow" is the axiom for prescribing such drugs for the patient with Alzheimer's disease. A starting dose of 0.5 mg of haloperidol (Haldol) often is adequate. Every patient who receives neuroleptic drugs should periodically be given a drug holiday (15 days without the drug), and the reason for its being prescribed must be clearly charted in every instance.

Behavior modification, as its name implies, seeks to change the objectionable behavior by either positively reinforcing acceptable alternative behavior or by negatively reinforcing unacceptable behavior. Negative reinforcement may take the form of "time-out," a period spent away from the activity of the institution or sitting in a chair in a corner. The plan for behavior modification should be carefully worked out with a professional who has the necessary skills for devising a good plan. The reader is referred to *Behavior Modification in Applied Settings*.

Restraints occasionally may be necessary, but, they should be used for short periods only and in emergency situations. Restraints often aggravate rather than alleviate aggressive behavior, since patients with Alzheimer's disease hate to be confined.

TREATING ALZHEIMER'S DISEASE WITH MEDICATION

Although a number of drugs are being investigated for treating Alzheimer's disease, none has yet proved to be effective and safe. However, it is probable that in the near future a drug or drugs that could be used to treat Alzheimer's disease will become available. To better understand the action of such drugs, it is important to know how impulses are transmitted to different parts of the brain and what happens in Alzheimer's disease.

When a nerve cell is stimulated, an electrical impulse is generated and moves along the nerve cell. When the impulse reaches the end of the nerve cell, it stimulates the production and release of chemical compounds called neurotransmitters (acetylcholine is an important one) into the synaptic cleft, the gap between two adjacent nerve cells. If enough acetylcholine is released, the nerve cell at the other end of the synapse is stimulated and the electrical impulse is transmitted to this cell. If insufficient acetylcholine is released, the neighboring cell is not stimulated and the electrical impulse dies out. Alzheimer's disease involves a deficiency of acetylcholine, and thus scientists have tried to find ways of increasing the brain stores of that neurotransmitter.

Acetylcholine cannot be given orally, because it is digested in the gastrointestinal tract before it can be absorbed. Even if given by injection, it has a number of unpleasant effects, including slowed heart rate and respiration, increased perspiration and often nausea, abdominal cramps, and a rise in body temperature.

Attempts have been made to give patients the precursors of acetylcholine, that is, substances the brain needs to produce acetylcholine. In fact, this theory forms the basis of a number of diets that are promoted as helping patients with Alzheimer's disease. These diets generally contain lettuce and other foods rich in lecithin, which is used to produce acetylcholine.

Unfortunately, although some anecdotal reports indicate that these diets help some patients, no convincing proof has emerged that patients benefit when put on such diets. Also, there is no convincing evidence of improvement in patients who are given orally large doses of lecithin, which can be bought over the counter in a number of health food stores. Currently, therefore, we do not believe that any benefit can be derived from altering the patient's diet to include lecithin precursors or by giving the patient large doses of lecithin orally. However, in the near future scientists probably will discover a compound that, when given orally, reaches the brain and increases the production of acetylcholine.

Because acetylcholine is broken down in the synapse, slowing the rate of breakdown may leave enough acetylcholine in the synapse to stimulate the neighboring nerve cell. This hypothesis has been tested and found to be correct. Indeed, when physostigmine, a drug that prevents destruction of acetylcholine, is injected intravenously in patients with Alzheimer's disease, mental functions improve significantly. Unfortunately, the improvement is short-lived and associated with such side effects as excessive salivation, nausea, vomiting, slowing of the heart and respiratory rates and in some instances convulsions. Furthermore, physostigmine must be given frequently because of its short duration of action.

In 1986 reports emerged of a drug that could be given orally and that had the same effects as physostigmine. The drug was known as tetra-hydroaminoacridine, and the preliminary results of its use in patients with Alzheimer's disease were thought to be excellent, with most patients improving significantly. However, later reports were not so encouraging, and the drug has been associated with a number of serious side effects.

Other efforts focused on bethanechol chloride, which has a chemical structure similar to that of acetylcholine. Researchers assumed that if bethanechol could be administered directly into the brains of patients with Alzheimer's disease, the patients' symptoms would improve. So a pump that could be surgically implanted was devised to deliver the drug into the brain. However, follow-up of patients who received this treatment showed no significant improvement, and bethanechol is no longer recommended for use in patients with Alzheimer's disease. Nonetheless, the means of administering it—a pump inserted surgically—could prove useful when an effective drug is discovered.

Ergoloid mesylate (Hydergine) a drug that is meant to enhance the metabolic activity of the brain, is often used in the management of patients with early Alzheimer's disease. The only convincing evidence is that it somewhat improves depression, confusion, unsociability, and lack of self-care; Some reports indicate that it also may improve dizziness. Ergoloid probably affects mostly the patient's mood and, to a lesser extent, behavior; it appears to have little effect on mental functions. However, since it may benefit some patients and is not associated with serious side effects, physicians frequently prescribe it for individuals with early Alzheimer's disease and other dementing illnesses. As a general rule, the earlier treatment is started, the more likely is the patient to respond favorably to this drug. If no change is noted in the patient's condition after 4 to 6 months of continuous treatment, the drug is unlikely to have an effect and continuing it would seem to be pointless.

A WORD OF CAUTION

Unquestionably, in the near future one or more drugs will become available specifically for treating Alzheimer's disease. Nevertheless, it is important to realize that no drug can be approved in the United States or any other Western country until it has been rigorously tested for effectiveness and safety. These are important safeguards intended to protect the public from false claims and potential side effects. Unfortunately, not all countries police drug production so stringently, and patients or their families may hear of a wonderful new "cure" that can be obtained only from a certain person and in a certain country.

Nurses and other health care professionals should be aware of any interest a patient or relative might show in such hoaxes, and they should advise the patient or family to discuss the matter with the patient's physician or to bring it to the attention of the local support group for relatives of patients with Alzheimer's disease.

BIBLIOGRAPHY

Becker R et al: Potential pharmacotherapy of Alzheimer disease. A comparison of various forms of physostigmine administration, Acta Neurol Scand (Suppl) 116:19-32, 1988.

Crook T: Pharmacotherapy of cognitive deficits in Alzheimer's disease and age-associated memory impairment, Psychopharmacol Bull 24(1):31-38, 1988.

Deutsch SI and Morihisa JM: Glutamatergic abnormalities in Alzheimer's disease and a rationale for clinical trials with L-glutamate, Clin Neuropharmacol 11(1):18-35, 1988.

Fisk AA: Management of Alzheimer's disease, Postgrad Med 73(4):237-241, 1983.

Gottlieb GL, McAllister TW, and Gur RC: Depot neuroleptics in the treatment of behavior disorders in patients with Alzheimer's disease, J Am Geriatr Soc 36:619-621, 1988.

Hamill RW et al: Neurodegenerative disorders and aging. Alzheimer's disease and Parkinson's disease—common ground, Ann NY Acad Sci 515:411-420, 1988.

Maletta GJ: Management of behavior problems in elderly patients with Alzheimer's disease and other dementias, Clin Geriatr Med (4):719-747, 1988.

Meyer JS et al: Improved cognition after control of risk factors for multiinfarct dementia, JAMA 256(16):2203-2209, 1986.

Mohs RC et al: Oral physostigmine treatment of patients with Alzheimer's disease, Am J Psychiatry 142(1):28-33, 1985.

Perry E: Acetylcholine and Alzheimer's disease, Br J Psychiatry 152:737-747, 1988.

Price DL et al: Neurobiological studies of transmitter systems in aging and in Alzheimer's–type dementia, Ann NY Acad Sci 47:35-51, 1985.

Reifler BV: Clinical problems in geriatric psychiatry. The relationship between dementia of the Alzheimer's type and depression, NC Med J 49(10):536-538, 1988.

Reynolds CF III et al: The nature and management of sleep/wake disturbance in Alzheimer's dementia, Psychopharmacol Bull 24(1):43-48, 1988.

Summers WK et al: Oral tetrahydroaminoacridine in long-term treatment of senile dementia, Alzheimer's type, N Engl J Med 316:1605-1606, 1987.

Teri L, Larson EB, and Reifler BV: Behavioral disturbance in dementia of the Alzheimer's type, J Am Geriatr Soc 36(1):1-6, 1988.

Thal LJ et al: Chronic oral physostigmine without lecithin improves memory in Alzheimer's disease, J Am Geriatr Soc 37(1):42-48, 1989.

Waters C: Cognitive enhancing agents: current status in the treatment of Alzheimer's disease, Can J Neurol Sci 15(3):249-256, 1988.

Winograd CH and Jarvik LF: Physician management of the demented patient, J Am Geriatr Soc 34:295-308, 1986.

Wragg RE and Jeste DV: Neuroleptics and alternative treatments. Management of behavioral symptoms and psychosis in Alzheimer's disease and related conditions, Psychiatr Clin North Am 11(1):195-213, 1988.

UNIT TWO
SPECIAL ISSUES IN CARE

5

Safety and accident prevention

L. Norman, M. Lancaster, and R. Hamdy

Patients with Alzheimer's disease are prone to a number of accidents. The type of accident and its prevention depend greatly on what stage of the disease the patient is in.

PATIENTS IN STAGE 1 (EARLY STAGE)
Driving a Car

Traffic accidents often are among the earliest signs that alert an individual's relatives to the fact that something is wrong with the person's mental functions. Common driving problems include becoming lost and failing to stop at traffic lights or stop or yield signs.

As was discussed in Chapter 1, a patient in stage 1 of Alzheimer's disease may appear normal or just "eccentric", (at least to people who do not know him), although there is definite memory impairment, as well as impairment in other cognitive fields. Because of this seeming normalcy, the decision whether to stop someone from driving is always a difficult one to make, especially since driving may represent the patient's only means of independence. Surprisingly also, many patients with early Alzheimer's disease can still drive themselves to the local shopping center or to relatives' or friends' homes; they do so almost automatically. Nevertheless, because these individuals have definite mental impairment and their reaction time is considerably slower than normal, they are a hazard to other drivers, to pedestrians, and to themselves.

Patients with Alzheimer's disease may forget the meaning of road signs, confuse the meaning of red and green traffic lights, incorrectly gauge the distance between vehicles, or simply forget which way to go. Any one of these mistakes could cause a serious accident.

Patients in the early stages of Alzheimer's disease also find it difficult to integrate and understand the meaning of a number of stimuli received simultaneously. As a result, they appear to be easily distracted, which is often a cause of traffic accidents. For instance, the patient may be distracted by road construction and may not notice that a traffic light has changed to red or that he is about to crash into the car in front of him.

Persuading a patient with Alzheimer's disease that he should not drive a car may be difficult. When explaining to the individual that he is no longer capable of driving, simply using specific details may not work; it may be necessary to hide the car keys. Also, having a physician tell the patient that he can no longer drive may be effective. As a last resort, the car may have to be sold or the engine altered so that it will not start (e.g., disconnecting the distributor).

Becoming Lost

Patients with Alzheimer's disease also frequently lose their way. They lose the ability to integrate various stimuli and to orient themselves and consequently often are unable to retrace their steps back home. In many instances individuals with Alzheimer's disease have taken a bus or train and been found wandering miles from home. Because of this tendency to become lost, these patients run the risk of being mugged or becoming victims of violence.

Patients with Alzheimer's disease appear to have a deep-rooted need to keep moving, a phenomenon that seems even more pronounced in the second stage of the disease. This raises the issue of somehow constraining the patient; yet it is another difficult decision whether to prevent him from leaving the house, particularly since this often increases his agitation and irritability.

Poor Judgment

In the first stage of Alzheimer's disease, patients may not be fully aware of some of the risks they take. For example, a patient may not remember to make sure that traffic is clear before crossing the street and consequently, may be hit by a car. Similarly, at home a patient may use a poorly balanced ladder to try to reach an object on a high shelf.

Gullibility

Because many patients in stage 1 are still relatively independent and able to communicate, it is not unusual for unscrupulous people and organizations to take advantage of their impaired mental functions. The patient may be approached by people who persuade him to part with his money or property, and the legal problems that could follow are very complex. Therefore, if the patient's judgment is felt to be poor, power of attorney probably should be granted to a more responsible person. It is also important to remember that individuals with Alzheimer's disease may invite strangers into their home, and these strangers may abuse the patient.

PATIENTS IN STAGE 2 (MIDDLE STAGE)

In the second stage, patients with Alzheimer's disease are easily recognized as having some mental abnormality, since mental functions are grossly impaired. If the patient is allowed to wander outside the house, he is likely to be involved in a car accident. The main accidents in the second stage of Alzheimer's disease are repeated falls and a number of personal injuries.

Repeated Falls

Repeated falls are common in older patients, particularly in patients with Alzheimer's disease. On average about half the falls are secondary to some intrinsic problem such as orthostatic hypotension, arrhythmias, Parkinson's disease, neuropathies, and epilepsy; the other half are caused by external factors such as poor lighting, a loose carpet, or awkwardly placed objects. Patients who cannot perceive their surroundings because of diminished vision or hearing are more likely to fall.

Besides all these factors, patients with Alzheimer's disease often take unnecessary risks. For instance, such a patient may place a chair atop a table and attempt to climb on both to reach an object on a high shelf; the results are often disastrous. Similarly, the patient may decide to paint a room, repair a window, or clean out the gutters and in the process may take risks that increase his chances of falling.

The patient with Alzheimer's disease reacts more slowly, which makes it difficult for him to regain his balance if he starts to fall. This slow reaction time is one reason it is so important to ensure that the patient's surroundings are free of any potential hazards that may cause falls. These hazards may include electrical wires, unevenness of the floor, throw rugs, and so forth.

Friends and family members who visit the patient should be reminded not to rearrange the furniture or place things on the floor. The patient cannot easily adapt to changes, and he performs best in surroundings that he knows well. When furniture or household items are moved, the patient may bump into them and fall.

Throw rugs are very dangerous to elderly people and especially to patients with Alzheimer's disease. Loose rugs are hazardous because the patient may catch his toe underneath the edge, trip, and fall, possibly suffering a broken hip. Rugs should be made slip-proof for everyone's safety, but particularly for that of elderly patients with Alzheimer's disease. Some throw rugs or decorative rugs that have been in place for many years may be precious to the family and may have a great sentimental value. They may also help with the patient's orientation by keeping the surroundings familiar. In these cases the rugs should be given nonslip backing, or the edges should be secured to the floor with nails or double-sided adhesive tape. Bulky rugs should be replaced by thinner ones that do not sit so high off the floor.

Removing obstacles from the common path of traffic throughout the house is important. If large pieces of furniture must remain where they are, any sharp edges or corners should be padded to prevent serious injury. All traffic pathways and rooms commonly used should be well lit. Bedrooms, bathrooms, hallways, and stairwells also require good lighting. Highly polished floors and direct sunlight into rooms should be avoided, since these produce glare, which older people find difficult to cope with. Glare can be reduced by using low-luster polishes on floors and by placing sheer curtains over windows.

Patients with Alzheimer's disease may not be able to gauge accurately the height of steps, curbs, and door thresholds; this often leads to falls. The edges of steps can be highlighted in a bright color to help draw the patient's attention to the steps, or barriers can be used to block stairways. However, the barriers should be high enough that the patient will not try to walk over them. Doors leading to basements should be kept locked.

Fire Hazards

Patients in stage 2 are also very likely to suffer personal injuries and are at risk of injuring or electrocuting themselves with electrical gadgets. Most of these accidents stem from the patient's poor memory. For example, deciding to cook a meal, the patient may turn on the gas oven but forget to light it. Or he may forget about the food he has put on the stove to cook.

Patients with Alzheimer's disease inadvertently pose frequent fire hazards, because they often do not appreciate the significance of many of their actions, and they can be easily distracted.

Electrical appliances, stoves, heaters, and matches pose particular dangers. Frequently the patient may turn on one of these appliances and leave it unattended. Changing or removing control knobs from stoves and heaters can help prevent patients from turning them on. Gas stoves are especially hazardous because the gas may be turned on but not lit; this can lead to gas poisoning or an explosion. Also, electrical outlets should be covered when not in use.

Bathing

Not uncommonly, patients with Alzheimer's disease are easily distracted while preparing to bathe. As a result, the faucet may be left on, and the patient may not realize that water has been overflowing the tub. Patients also may either scald themselves with bath water that is too hot, or expose themselves to hypothermia with water that is too cold.

Similarly, patients may forget or be unable to turn the heat on or may not realize that although the heat is on, the house will not warm up with the windows open. They also may be unable to appreciate the need to dress appropriately. These patients tend to go outside inappropriately dressed and are likely to suffer from inclement weather. Hypothermia appears to be a significant risk in patients with Alzheimer's disease.

Poisoning

Accidents with detergents, such as spilling some compounds on oneself, or swallowing household cleaning fluids, are more likely to happen to patients with Alzheimer's disease.

In cases of food poisoning, the patient's diminished senses of smell and taste may prevent him from noticing a strong smell or "off" taste in spoiled food. Thus these patients may not be able to distinguish food that has gone bad from wholesome food, and they are much more at risk of developing food poisoning. Similarly, these patients may forget to return food to the refrigerator.

Medication

Patients with Alzheimer's disease are likely either to take the wrong medicine or to take the correct medicine but at the wrong time; they also may take too much. One of the authors had a patient in the second stage of Alzheimer's disease who took his sleeping medication first thing in the morning and his diuretics the last thing before going to bed. Consequently, the patient tended to be lethargic and sleepy most of the day and incontinent and fully awake at night. It had been generally assumed that these two conditions were the result of Alzheimer's disease, when in fact they were caused by the inappropriately taken medication.

The patient must not have unlimited access to medications. He may take a sleeping tablet, then forget that he took it and a few minutes later, take another. This sequence may be repeated several times, until the patient has taken an overdose of hypnotic medication. A number of gadgets can be used to prevent the patient from taking more medication than required. For instance, all the day's medication may be placed in a small compartment of a special container, while the main compartment containing the rest of the medication is made inaccessible. A note may be left in the container saying that, since no tablets are left, the patient must have taken his medication for the day and should not try to take more. This may prevent the patient from becoming agitated at not being able to take additional medication.

The same risk of overdose may apply to a patient who is in pain, who has analgesic preparations at hand, and who tries to relieve the pain. Because his memory is poor, he may forget having taken an analgesic tablet and thus may take a large quantity of this medication. Overdosage of many preparations such as hypotensive medications and medications that act on the heart may be associated with serious side effects. Therefore no medication should be left lying around. As much as possible, the patient should be given his medication on a day-to-day basis.

It is wise to have the caregiver take charge of all the patient's medication and administer the medication as prescribed. The caregiver must to be instructed on how and when to give the medication, as well as the common side effects. In this way the caregiver will be prepared and able to consult with the doctor should any side effects occur.

Wandering

Wandering is a problem many caregivers must face with patients with Alzheimer's disease. Nursing homes with special units for these patients have an advantage, because they usually have an area that is locked for safety yet allows the patients to move about freely. Although the patient should be allowed as much independence as possible, the prevention of accidents caused by wandering outside the house must be considered when it is no longer safe for the patient to be out alone. Doors leading to the outside should be kept locked. Often simply changing to a new type of lock that the patient is not familiar with can solve the problem. If it does not, deadbolt locks requiring keys should be installed.

Regular door handles can be replaced with child-proof models that require a combination of actions to turn the handle. The patient with Alzheimer's disease probably would not be able to figure out the sequence necessary to open the door. Alarm systems on doors can also be helpful. These systems allow the door to be opened but signal the caregiver that the patient is going outside. Sometimes just the alarm would be enough to scare the patient off, so that he closes the door and does not go out. Many types of door alarms are available, and they vary in sophistication and cost. It is wise to shop around to find the system best suited to the patient, the caregiver, and the budget. Many nursing homes use alarm systems on the outside doors of buildings.

If the patient can go outside, fencing in the yard may be added protection. This allows the patient to get some fresh air and exercise in an enclosed, safe area. The yard should be kept clear of branches or other objects that might cause harm. Additionally, the patient should have adequate identification. A bracelet or locket can contain the information on whom to contact if the patient wanders away from home. The family should have a recent photograph of the patient that can be given to the neighbors or police if a search should become necessary. An identifying bracelet or necklace is also useful for informing whoever finds the patient about the disease and associated confusion. Lastly, neighbors and friends should be told of the patient's problem so that they can notify the caregiver if they find the patient wandering away from home. Also, the phone numbers of the police department and the neighbors should be kept handy.

Some patients will not go outside unless they are wearing their favorite jacket or shoes or are carrying their purse or wallet. This is probably a lifelong habit that the patient with Alzheimer's disease has maintained. Putting these articles out of sight until they are needed can help prevent the patient from wandering. It may be necessary to camouflage the door, as it may be a source of frustration to the patient. Pull-down shades or portable, decorative screens can effectively disguise the exit.

Pica

Pica is the craving and eating of unusual foods or substances, a trait not uncommon among patients with Alzheimer's disease. Because of this tendency, cleaning products constitute another area in which accident prevention is necessary. Two characteristics that patients with Alzheimer's disease sometimes have are an active appetite and an inquisitive nature. Although the patient may not gain weight, his appetite is good, and because he may no longer recognize which things are appropriate to eat, he may pick up some items as soap, cigarettes, and flowers and put them in his mouth. Thus cleaning products, medication, and all poisonous substances must be kept safely locked up. Mouth-washes and soaps should also be kept out of sight; although not poisonous, they can make a person very ill if taken in large amounts.

PATIENTS IN STAGE 3 (LATE STAGE)

In the third stage, the patient has a number of physical disabilities in addition to his mental impairment. Because of this, he is much more at risk of falling, becoming incontinent of urine, developing decubiti, and becoming dehydrated. Furthermore, because of his agitation, physical restraints are often applied.

Restraints

Physical restraints or restraint by means of drugs are sometimes used to ensure the patient's safety. The objective in using restraints is to protect the patient from falls and self-injury. Because the use of restraints conflicts with the overall treatment goal of maintaining the patient's independence, all alternative measures for safety should be exhausted before restraints are prescribed. Restraints should never be seen as the first or definitive solution to a safety problem and should not be used solely for the caregiver's convenience. In an institutional setting, it must also be remembered that, should a physician have to order restraints, the need for them must be clearly documented in the nursing notes.

Whenever a restraint is used, the goal is to eliminate it as soon as possible. Success in achieving this goal is measured by how quickly this can be accomplished. It must be remembered that restraints restrict the patient's movement and deny his independence and sense of freedom.

A common, unwanted side effect of restraints, especially when used with patients with Alzheimer's disease is aggressive, agitated behavior. Often the patient does not comprehend the reason for the restraint and begins to fight. He may think he is being tied down or punished. Conversely, some patients may exhibit regressive behavior and retreat further into isolation by not interacting. In either case the patient's confusion, isolation, and dependence will probably increase. If this occurs, engaging the patient in some activity and using therapeutic touch can help decrease agitation by distracting his attention from the restraints.

Many types of restraints are available: vests, wrist and ankle restraints, bar restraints, and belts. Each type has advantages and disadvantages, which should be considered when selecting the most appropriate one to meet the patient's needs.

Vest restraints are used frequently because they allow free movement of the arms and legs while supporting the upper body. This type of restraint is particularly useful for patients who tend to lean forward and are at risk of falling out of a wheelchair. Vest restraints can also be effective for patients who try to climb out of bed. A disadvantage to this restraint is that the patient can slide down and wiggle his way out of the vest. This can be dangerous if the restraint becomes caught underneath the chin and lodges around the neck; the patient is in effect hanging himself.

A patient can get out of a restraint even if it is correctly applied. By no means should the restraint be considered a sure safeguard against falls and accidents. The patient in restraint should be checked frequently to ensure that the restraint remains in place and that circulation and respiratory effort are not restricted. The patient's needs for toileting, food, fluid, and activity must also be met by releasing the restraints every 2 or 3 hours. All checks on the patient should be recorded in the nursing notes or in a flow sheet.

Any restraint must always be secured to a stable object. Restraints for bed patients should be secured to the bed frame and not to the side rail. Additionally, the patient should be able to roll from side to side in a vest restraint. Restraints for a patient in a wheelchair should never be fastened to a moveable part of the chair. Belt restraints can be securely fastened underneath the seat of the wheelchair. This type of restraint is best used with patients who only need reminding to call for assistance when they want to get up.

Side rails are a form of restraint that helps to remind the patient to stay in bed. When side rails are used, the bed should always be in the low position. If the patient decides to climb over the side rails and the bed is in the high position, the added distance that the patient falls can significantly increase injury. It is probably wise to use a vest restraint in conjunction with side rails for patients with Alzheimer's disease. Because their judgment and reasoning are impaired, they frequently do not understand the need for side rails and will try to climb over them.

If the patient is physically capable of walking, placing the bed in the low position and keeping the side rails lowered is probably the safest bed position for the patient. Most patients who had climbed over side rails or had fallen from bed reported that they were trying to get to the bathroom. *It is vital that the caregiver remember to attend frequently to the need for elimination.*

Arm, leg, or wrist restraints are seldom used. They should be used only when agitation is severe and this is the only method available to keep the patient from harming himself. Also, this type of restraint should be used only for short periods. Medications frequently are used in combination with arm, leg, or wrist restraints. If the patient requires this type of combined restraint, he must be assessed every hour and this assessment must be documented. Because arm or leg restraints severely restrict movement, more ethical and legal implications come into play. Hand mittens, which allow free movement, can be used instead of wrist restraints for patients who pull out their intravenous lines or feeding tubes.

The use of restraints is a controversial issue. Each state and local institution must have a policy outlining the requirements and procedures for using physical restraints, and each situation and patient must be analyzed individually. Health care workers must be made more aware that the use of restraints affects behavior. The patient's safety and well-being must be weighed against the risks and side effects of restraints; and the goal of using restraints for the least amount of time possible must always be kept in mind.

SUMMARY

Safety and accident prevention for patient's with Alzheimer's disease pose many difficulties for the caregiver. Being aware of potential hazards and realizing that the patient can no longer be responsible for his own safety is the first step in preventing accidents. Providing a safe environment, either at home or in the nursing home, can help lessen the strain on caregivers. Considerable patience and creativity are required to make an environment safe yet stimulating for patients with Alzheimer's disease.

BIBLIOGRAPHY

Bastow MD, Rawlings J, and Allison SP: Undernutrition, hypothermia, and injury in elderly women with fractured femur: an injury response to altered metabolism?, Lancet 1(8317):143-146, 1983.

Brody ED et al: Predictors of falls among institutionalized women with Alzheimer's disease, J Am Geriatr Soc 32(12):877-882, 1984.

Buchner DM and Larson EB: Transfer bias and the association of cognitive impairment with falls, J Gen Intern Med 3(3):254-259, 1988.

Klenerman L et al: Bringing gait analysis out of the laboratory and into the clinic, Age and Ageing 17(6):397-400, 1988.

Koller WC et al: Falls and Parkinson's disease, Clin Neuropharmacol 12(2):98-105, 1989.

Lucas-Blaustein MJ et al: Driving in patients with dementia, J Am Geriatr Soc 36(12):1087-1091, 1988.

Mossey JM: Social and psychologic factors related to falls among the elderly, Clin Geriatr Med 1(3)541-553, 1985.

6

Hygiene and the patient with Alzheimer's disease

L. Norman and M. Lancaster

One of the first signs of impairment usually noticed in patients with Alzheimer's disease is a change in hygiene or grooming habits. Basic hygiene practices are ingrained in long-term memory but require the use of short-term memory to initiate the actions. Patients will forget to bathe, change clothes, or use the bathroom. These tasks appear simple but actually require a number of sequential actions to complete them. For example, a patient may remember to take a bath but forget what to do first. Reminding him of the task may not be enough to help him accomplish it.

Caregivers must not only be attuned to the patient's general hygienic needs, but also must determine the specific area of impairment so as to give the correct assistance. Completing the task for the patient may not be the correct measure. If the patient can complete his hygienic care by means of simple reminders or aids, he will remain independent longer and increase his sense of self-esteem and his feeling of control. If the patient is not allowed to participate in a task, such as dressing, he will forget how to perform the task and will lose the ability to perform it in the future. *It is most important to remember that, for the patient with Alzheimer's disease, once a skill is lost, it is virtually impossible to regain.*

Assessment of the patient's skill level is very important. In accomplishing a task of basic hygiene, breaking it down into steps is helpful. For example, the patient may be able to brush his teeth himself if the toothpaste is placed on the brush for him and the brush is set next to the cold water faucet. Simply instructing the patient to brush his teeth may not work. Assessing the patient's skills and areas of impairment, breaking down a task into steps, and assisting only in the impaired areas will help keep the patient functioning independently longer.

MOUTH CARE

Patients with Alzheimer's disease often neglect daily cleansing of the mouth. If the patient does not perform this task it is extremely important for the caregiver to do it. Even if the patient has no natural teeth or dentures, the gums, cheeks, and tongue should be cleaned. Improper or inadequate mouth care can result in serious problems with both teeth and gums. The gums will quickly become irritated and inflamed, resulting in pain, exposure of the root of the tooth, and a site for infection. Build-up of food deposits on the teeth can lead to cavities. In addition, a mouth that is not properly cleaned causes bad breath and therefore a decrease in self-esteem.

Brushing one's teeth requires remembering where the bathroom is located, how to open the toothpaste tube, how to squeeze the tube to put the toothpaste on the toothbrush, how to hold the toothbrush, which water control to use and how to turn it on, what motion to use to brush the teeth, and the other steps necessary to complete the task. A patient who forgets one step, such as the location of the toothpaste, may not be able to complete the task. However, simply locating the toothpaste may be all that he needs to be able to brush his teeth. The patient should be observed to see if he is properly cleansing his mouth and where assistance may be needed.

The care of dentures requires a totally different set of skills in patients with Alzheimer's disease. Patients often misplace their dentures or clean them incorrectly, if at all. The patient should be encouraged to use his dentures to improve chewing ability, speech, and looks. Dentures should be removed at least daily and scrubbed with a soft brush and cleanser. While effervescent cleansing tablets are commonly used, they do not clean the dentures as well as a brush and cleanser. Food particles should be removed from the teeth and the top and bottom of the plate brushed to remove any food, mucus, or adhesive. The patient's mouth should be rinsed well or swabbed out while the dentures are out. If the dentures are going to be out for any length of time, they should be stored in water. The denture wearer's mouth should be inspected periodically for signs of irritation.

Periodic examinations by a dentist/hygienist should be continued as long as possible. Some dentists will make house calls or trips to nursing homes if the patient is unable to come to their office. Adaptive devices are also available to help hold the patient's mouth open so that proper cleaning can be performed. Even if the patient is no longer taking food or fluid by mouth or is being fed through a tube, the mouth should not be neglected.

BATHING

A bath or shower seems to be the first area that produces significant resistance in the patient with Alzheimer's disease. Since the sense of smell may be decreased in Alzheimer's disease, the patient may not remember why he needs to bathe or that he needs to undress to bathe. He may also fear what will happen to him if he is undressed. The sensation of the shower may be associated with standing in the rain rather than bathing. Sitting in the bathtub may be perceived as being "punished." Reminding the patient that this is a bath or shower is helpful but may not be effective. Having the patient sit in a shower chair or bath seat may help him accept the procedure. If the patient becomes combative or extremely agitated in preparing for the bath or shower, it is better to delay the activity until he can accept it. Establishing a routine of bathing on specific days can help with acceptance of the bath. Sometimes the patient will accept help from an outside caregiver more readily than from a family member. If the patient becomes agitated about having a bath when this is requested by a family member, a home health assistant may be necessary for hygienic care.

In the early stages of Alzheimer's disease, reminding the patient of the bath and drawing the water may be all that is necessary to complete the task. The patient must be assessed for his ability to distinguish the hot and cold water faucets and for his knowledge of how to regulate water temperature. He may turn on the hot water once in the bath or shower and receive a burn. Turning down the temperature on the hot water heater may be necessary to prevent burns, since patients with Alzheimer's disease often lose their ability to distinguish hot and cold.

An elderly patient usually does not need a complete bath every day; once or twice a week is sufficient for cleansing of the skin. The aging process causes the skin to lose its elasticity, and irritation and injury result if a person bathes too frequently. Secretion of oil and sebum also decrease with age, thereby decreasing the need for frequent bathing. The skin becomes dry, thin, and fragile and can be easily injured by too much manipulation. Too frequent bathing may also lead to itching from dryness and may deceive the caretakers into believing that even more vigorous washing is needed. The patients underarms and genital area should be washed regularly, but a bath or shower should be limited to once or twice a week.

Because the skin of elderly patients is so fragile, soaps must be chosen with care. Mild soaps and emollients in the bathwater help decrease dryness of the skin. Care must be taken when assisting the patient out of the tub when emollients are used, because they make the tub or shower surface slippery. Bath oils should be added to the bathwater after the person is in the tub, since this allows the oil to seal in moisture the skin has absorbed. Drying the skin, particularly any skin folds, is important. Unscented powders or cornstarch may be needed to keep these areas dry. The skin can break down if these areas are not kept dry. Inspecting the skin regularly is important, particularly for patients who can still bathe themselves. A decrease in pain perception may accompany the aging process, and the patient may be unaware that he has an area of skin breakdown. Routine inspection will alert the caregiver to areas that need attention before breakdown actually occurs.

DRESSING

Inappropriate dressing may be one of the first signs of Alzheimer's disease noticeable to family and friends. The patient may not coordinate colors, may put a shirt on backward, or may fasten buttons in the wrong order. The act of dressing is as complex a task as the other hygiene practices.

In the early stages of Alzheimer's disease, the patient's closet and dresser drawers should be organized into colors and outfits. This can help eliminate the need to remember, for example, that the red blouse goes with the blue skirt. Catastrophic reactions often occur when patients become frustrated while trying to coordinate colors or choose clothing.

As the disease progresses, the patient loses fine motor coordination. He may not be able to manipulate small buttons, hooks, or zippers. Using Velcro closures or long, large zippers will help him continue to dress himself. Clothes that fasten in the front are easier for the patient to manipulate than those that have to be pulled over the head. The patient may become agitated by pulling a shirt or dress over the head, because he may feel threatened by this movement. Stiffening of the muscles makes dressing harder for the patient with Alzheimer's disease. His clothing must be loose to compensate for the decreased flexibility in the arms and legs. Clothes with elastic waistbands, such as jogging pants, are easier to get on and off and help the patient to remain independent for a longer period. The clothing should also be of soft, wash-and-wear fabric to decrease the burden on the caregiver in keeping the patient's clothes clean and neat.

Increasing agitation may be noticed in the clothes that the patient chooses to wear. He may put on several layers of clothes as he becomes more confused. It may be that he is searching for the correct thing to wear, or he may have forgotten to remove the first items. The layering of clothes should be explored further with the patient, as he actually may be expressing another need such as pain, hunger, or frustration.

TOILETING

A patient with Alzheimer's disease may need to be reminded to go to the bathroom frequently to empty his bladder. He may not pay attention to the feeling of bladder fullness or may recognize that his bladder is full but forget where the bathroom is located. It is not uncommon for these patients to become incontinent, and establishing a schedule of toileting throughout the day helps to keep them dry. The causes, treatment, and management of incontinence is discussed further in Chapters 10 and 11.

Maintaining normal bowel function in the patient with Alzheimer's disease often takes creativity and the advice of health professionals. Changes in the digestive system that occur with age cause the older person to be prone to constipation. In addition, the patient with Alzheimer's disease may not "feel" the need for a bowel movement, may forget how to have a bowel movement, or will defecate at inappropriate times and in inappropriate places. Taking the patient to the bathroom at the same time every day and having him sit on the toilet is the first step in establishing a regular bowel maintenance program and prevention of accidents. The patient should be observed to identify the time of day when his bowels normally act. Sometimes a cup of hot liquid, such as coffee, 30 minutes before toileting can help to stimulate bowel action.

The patient should be kept as active as possible because this facilitates bowel motion. Adequate fluid and fiber in the patient's diet help keep the stool soft and guard against constipation. Fiber can be added to the diet in the form of cereals, muffins, and whole-grain bread. If laxatives with fiber are used, increase amount of water the patient drinks each day.

Lightly massaging the lower abdomen can sometimes stimulate a bowel movement. As increasing difficulty is encountered, simply inserting a glycerin suppository and having the patient sit on the toilet often results in a bowel movement. Stronger laxatives, enemas, and suppositories should be used only after the above methods have been tried.

The debilitated patient need not have a bowel movement every day. However, he should have a movement at least every third day. One or two suppositories can be used every third day to empty the bowels of persons who can no longer have a spontaneous bowel movement. If a patient begins to have small, diarrhetic stools, leakage of small amounts of feces, or complains of abdominal cramping, he should be checked for a fecal impaction, which is often the cause of these symptoms. A laxative or stool softener frequently will help remove the impaction. If not, the patient may need an enema.

Loss of bowel control is traumatic, health professionals can help devise a management plan. Incontinence pads help keep bed linen and chair covers clean. For more active patients, the new incontinence pants have eased care and made life more pleasant for the patient and caregiver.

OTHER HYGIENIC TASKS

Eventually the patient will need help with other tasks that are part of overall hygiene. Fingernails and toenails should be trimmed and filed regularly, and they should be kept short to prevent injury from scratching. Toenails should be trimmed straight across, whereas fingernails are rounded on the ends. The nails should be cleaned regularly to remove dirt, feces, oils, and dead skin, which accumulate under the nail. An occasional manicure and polishing would be a real treat for a patient.

Also, the patient's ears should not be neglected. The outside part of the ear can easily be washed with a cloth wrapped over a finger. Swabs can be used, but the tip should always be visible (i.e., the ear canal should not be entered). Improper use of swabs serves only to push wax farther into the ear. Aging causes the wax in the ears to become dryer and more easily packed down, which can result in substantial hearing loss. If the patient seems to be having more difficulty hearing, he should be seen by a physician. The ear canals may need to be professionally cleaned to remove the impacted wax.

Shaving is another task that requires safety and supervision. Once the patient's coordination and judgment are impaired, an electric razor can be used to keep him independent and safe in the activity. Beards and mustaches need not be shaved, but they should be kept short, neat, and clean. Because food particles often become embedded in a beard, it should be thoroughly cleansed after each meal. If an electric razor is used, shaving should be supervised to ensure that electrical safety practices are followed (not shaving with water in the sink, correct plugging in and unplugging of the cord). Rechargeable battery-operated razors can be used to avoid the above hazards. Applying a small amount of after-shave can help the patient feel good about himself. For women patients, cream depilatories can be used on legs and underarms. A skin patch test should be performed before the product is used to note any sensitivity to it.

Women patients who previously have worn makeup should be encouraged to continue the practice, as this can give their self-esteem a boost. The patient should be supervised when applying makeup as it often is done inappropriately. The patient may "cake on" the makeup or apply it in a patchy fashion. She may forget to cleanse the skin before more makeup is applied and may end up with layers of cosmetics on her face, which can result in facial skin problems. Limiting the choice of colors to two tones can prevent indecision or the choice of a "totally wrong" color.

Hygienic practices may seem simple and well ingrained in everyone. Yet each task requires decisions, judgment, coordination, and memory. Each of these abilities is impaired in the patient with Alzheimer's disease, and consequently his caregivers must continually assess his abilities and provide guidance and assistance as needed. Helping the patient to complete each task with the least amount of assistance helps to improve his self-esteem and body image.

BIBLIOGRAPHY

Evans LK: Nursing the hospitalized dementia patient, J Adv Med Surg Nurs 1(2):18-31, 1989.

Teri L, Larson EB, and Reifler BV: Behavioral disturbance in dementia of the Alzheimer's type, J Am Geriatr Soc 36(1):1-6, 1988.

7

Nutrition and Alzheimer's disease

R. Hamdy and R. Acuff

It is rare to see an obese patient with Alzheimer's disease. Indeed, several surveys have revealed that most, if not all patients with Alzheimer's disease appear to be underweight and malnourished compared to patients who do not have the disease. Even when compared to patients with other dementing illnesses, those with Alzheimer's disease appear to be consistently underweight. It is therefore unlikely that this weight loss is the result only of a poor dietary intake secondary to the patient's mental impairment and his forgetting to eat regularly. Furthermore, patients with Alzheimer's disease appear to "fade away" gradually. These observations have led some investigators to suspect that Alzheimer's disease may be caused by malnutrition, and a number of research projects have been undertaken to discover whether this is the case.

IS ALZHEIMER'S DISEASE CAUSED BY NUTRITIONAL DEFICIENCIES?

Physicians and researchers have known for some time that deficiencies of certain vitamins, such as vitamin B_{12}, may lead to impaired mental functions and even to full-blown dementia. It therefore was suggested that Alzheimer's disease may be caused by some nutritional deficiency. A few of the initial studies appeared to produce promising results.

Several investigators demonstrated independently that cachexia (severe weight loss associated with dehydration) was found almost uniformly among patients with advanced Alzheimer's disease. It was then established that the blood levels of some nutritional parameters were much lower in patients with Alzheimer's disease than in patients with other types of dementia. Furthermore, some investigators were able to demonstrate not only a positive correlation between the reduced blood levels and the degree of mental impairment, but also a certain improvement after administering the nutritional substances that were deficient. The scene was set to determine the lack of which particular nutritional element leads to Alzheimer's disease if the patient does not consume it.

Another major step in this direction was the discovery that patients with Alzheimer's disease have reduced quantities of certain neurotransmitters in the brain. Of particular significance was the finding that the concentrations of acetylcholine and serotonin specifically were much less in patients with Alzheimer's disease than in those with other dementing illnesses. Of even greater significance was the apparent improvement of some patients when given food substances that eventually were transformed into acetylcholine and serotonin in the brain. These findings eventually led to the development of certain diets that were thought to benefit patients with Alzheimer's disease and to the hypothesis that Alzheimer's disease is caused by malnutrition.

More investigators became interested and involved in studying the relationship between Alzheimer's disease and malnutrition. The tools they used became more accurate and sensitive, and at the same time it became possible to diagnose Alzheimer's disease with a fair degree of accuracy (ranging from 80% to 90%). The scene was set to confirm unequivocally the relationship between inadequate dietary intake, or malnutrition, and Alzheimer's disease.

Unfortunately, the results from many subsequent studies were disappointing. Although it could not be denied that patients with Alzheimer's disease were significantly underweight when compared to other patients of similar age, sex, and even with other types of dementias, this weight loss could not be accounted for by any definite deficit in food intake.

It was then suggested that perhaps patients with Alzheimer's disease have an adequate food intake but are unable to absorb the food through the gastrointestinal tract. More research was done to study the gastrointestinal absorption of various food products in patients with Alzheimer's disease, but these results also were disappointing. Patients with Alzheimer's disease did not have any identifiable deficit in the absorption of food through the gastrointestinal tract. Finally, several well-designed studies that were rigorously conducted failed to demonstrate any significant relationship between Alzheimer's disease and inadequate nutritional intake or inadequate absorption of food from the gastrointestinal tract.

Currently the consensus is that there is no evidence that Alzheimer's disease is caused by nutritional deficiencies. Similarly, there is no scientific evidence that altering a patient's diet will improve his condition. Although many anecdotal cases may exist, any apparent improvement in the patient's condition is probably caused by some other factor or is a chance occurrence.

IS ALZHEIMER'S DISEASE CAUSED BY FOOD POISONING?

Some researchers, instead of looking for evidence of malnutrition, began looking for evidence of food toxicity. In other words, they stipulated that perhaps patients develop Alzheimer's disease because they continuously eat something that may be detrimental to the brain.

Aluminum and Alzheimer's Disease

Aluminum, one of the most abundant metals in the Earth's crust, has been found in some regions of the brains of patients with Alzheimer's disease. Thus some researchers believed that the disease may be a form of aluminum poisoning. They proposed that, as this metal is deposited in the brain, it destroys the brain cells. This theory has caused some concern, especially among individuals who use aluminum cookware. However, several reports have indicated that dietary aluminum consumption from cookware is relatively small and insignificant. Also, in most cases involving aluminum deposits in the brain, the patients were taking some medication containing this metal or were undergoing renal hemodialysis; the fluid used for the dialysis is rich in aluminum. If a correlation does exist between aluminum consumption and the development or progression of Alzheimer's disease, the source of contamination is not likely to be aluminum cookware.

Finally, many patients with Alzheimer's disease do not have aluminum deposits in the brain. Indeed, the evidence currently available does not suggest that aluminum plays any role in the development of Alzheimer's disease.

MALNUTRITION AND ALZHEIMER'S DISEASE
The Role of Food and Drink in Society

Although malnutrition is unlikely to be the cause of Alzheimer's disease, many patients with Alzheimer's disease do become both malnourished and dehydrated. There are several reasons for this that must be considered in the context of the normal person's average food and fluid intake.

Fluid intake

The average worker (Mr. Jones) has a cup of coffee with breakfast. More coffee during the morning at work, and almost always something to drink with lunch. In the afternoon he will drink more liquids, coffee and some other beverage will accompany dinner, and many individuals have a nightcap before retiring. It is important to realize that most of these fluids were consumed not because the person was thirsty, but to comply with certain social rituals, which may have evolved specifically to avoid the risk of becoming dehydrated.

When the average person retires from his job, he won't have to get up early any more. He won't have to rush his morning cup of coffee at breakfast before going to work, and as time passes, he tends to combine breakfast and coffee break into one session. He'll still have his midday meal but will only occasionally go out for lunch. Also, instead of having tea or coffee at two different times in the afternoon (once at work and once on his return home), he'll probably content himself with only one drink. As time passes, he may even combine the afternoon coffee with his supper. The number of times he goes out to eat or drink will be curtailed.

In other words, when Mr. Jones stops working and retires, he is reducing his opportunities of drinking fluids by about half, and he will rely more often on his sense of thirst to drink rather than having drinks to comply with social rituals.

Another factor of equal importance is that the sense of thirst tends to diminish and be dulled as a person ages. When Mr. Jones was 20 years younger, whenever his body needed fluids, he felt thirsty and drank. Now Mr. Jones' body may be desperately in need of fluids, yet he does not feel thirsty. So he gradually becomes dehydrated without noticing it. If in addition he has Alzheimer's disease, he may totally ignore his sense of thirst or hunger and become both dehydrated and malnourished. This is especially likely to occur when the biological clock is not functioning adequately and when the day/night pattern is reversed.

A person drinks for only two reasons, because he is thirsty or because society expects him to drink. It is indeed remarkable how all civilizations rotate around meals and drinks. Patients with Alzheimer's disease, therefore, are particularly at risk of neither drinking nor eating sufficiently.

Other factors also make elderly patients prone to becoming dehydrated more rapidly than younger people. When the human body is deprived of fluids, the kidneys tend to reabsorb a large quantity of water from the urine, which becomes more concentrated. In fact, this is sometimes used as a test of renal function (urine concentration test). As the kidneys age, they cannot concentrate the urine much; as a result, larger volumes of urine are formed, regardless of whether the person is dehydrated. Unless these quantities are replaced by drinking, the person may become dehydrated because he is eliminating more fluid than he is taking in. This is more likely to happen if the person's sense of thirst is dulled and if there are no special incentives to drink. Diuretic drugs used to treat heart failure also may cause dehydration.

An elderly person risks becoming dehydrated because he has fewer opportunities for drinking, because the sense of thirst often is dulled, because the kidneys often cannot concentrate the urine, because the individual may be taking diuretic drugs, and finally, if he has Alzheimer's disease, he may not be able to appreciate the need to drink and eat. Thus the caregiver must be aware of these facts and ensure that the patient is not becoming dehydrated.

Food intake

Malnutrition may be caused by other factors. For example, socio-economic reasons may force an older person to eat a less nutritious diet. Not only is the total number of calories consumed reduced, but often more carbohydrates and fats are consumed, whereas less protein is eaten. Bread and margarine are cheaper than meat and fish. Many elderly people prefer food that is rich in carbohydrates and fat to that rich in protein, since the former is easier to chew. Problems with teeth and dentures are common in the elderly.

Taste perception may be less sensitive in old age, and this in turn may make most food unpalatable and may blunt the person's appetite. The sense of taste is very dependent on the sense of smell, which is often diminished in Alzheimer's disease. Most of the pleasure derived from food depends on its presentation and appearance, yet failing eyesight resulting from cataracts, glaucoma, or other eye diseases distorts the appearance of food. Many other factors may lead the older person to consume a less nutritious diet, including depression, loneliness, and certain medications.

These altered dietary habits may occur some time before Alzheimer's disease becomes manifest, and they may become pronounced after the diagnosis is made. Of particular relevance is the lack of vitamins and minerals in the patient's diet. Many elderly people live on their own and must rely on social services or neighbors and friends to provide them with cooked meals. Not infrequently, these meals are reheated several times. With each reheating cycle more vitamins are destroyed, so that finally, when the elderly person consumes the food, the vitamin nutritional value is very much reduced.

Classification of Food Substances

Food substances customarily are divided into several categories: energy-producing substances (carbohydrates, proteins, and fats); vitamins (i.e., vitamins A, B, C, D, E, and K); minerals (i.e., sodium, potassium, calcium, iodine, magnesium, manganese, and iron); dietary fiber (cellulose); and water. To help determine the amount from each of these categories that a person requires each day to remain healthy, minimum recommended daily dietary allowances have been developed.

The Recommended Daily Dietary Allowance (RDA) has been primarily developed by examining the nutrient needs of young, healthy adults and extrapolating these results to the very young and old. This is unfortunate for both groups, because of the non-homogeneous nature of the very young and old. It can therefore, be stated that the nutritional needs of the elderly are uncertain.

Energy-producing substances

Proteins. The body uses proteins for growth and for regeneration of destroyed cells; proteins also play a vital role in tissue repair. It is a well-known fact that after surgery, patients with an adequate protein intake fare much better than those whose intake is inadequate.

The current recommended daily allowance is 0.8 g of protein per kilogram of body weight each day for individuals over 51 years of age. It has been suggested in this age group that 12% or more of total energy intake should be in the form of protein.

Carbohydrates. Carbohydrates are good sources of energy, which is why some sportsmen and bicycle riders in particular have occasional sips of a sweet drink while exercising. However, if more carbohydrates than the body needs are consumed, the excess is changed to fat. Sources of carbohydrates include sugar and most starchy substances, bread, potatoes, rice, and macaroni.

Fats. Fats can be either saturated (e.g., animal fats such as butter or lard) or unsaturated (oils and fats derived from plants, such as olive or corn oil and margarine). This difference is important, because the saturated fats are likely to precipitate arteriosclerosis, to increase the amount of cholesterol and triglycerides in the blood, and to be quite harmful. The unsaturated fats (especially the polyunsaturated ones such as vegetable oils) not only are less likely to lead to arteriosclerosis, but also reduce the levels of cholesterol and triglycerides. They therefore have a protective action in the body. Moreover, if saturated and unsaturated fats are eaten at the same time, less of each will be absorbed from the gastrointestinal tract.

It is important to try to prevent arteriosclerosis from developing and, if it is already present, to try to reduce its rate of progress. Although arteriosclerosis is not the cause of Alzheimer's disease, it is probably responsible for the second most common cause of dementing illnesses: multiinfarct dementia.

To prevent arteriosclerosis or to slow its progress, the amount of saturated fats in food should be reduced. This can be accomplished in several ways. First, lean meat should be chosen, since it contains less fat; thus chicken is better than pork or beef.

Second, the amount of fat in meat can be reduced further by discarding as much of the visible fat as possible. This can be done before cooking by cutting away all visible fat around the meat; it can also be done during cooking by removing the fat produced in the process, (for instance, while roasting meat). Third, cooking is better done using polyunsaturated fats rather than saturated fat; butter, lard, and suet should be avoided. Vegetable oil and margarine are recommended.

Fourth, a person should not eat any visible fat (e.g., the bacon rind). Fifth, rich sauces, full fat cheeses, and cream should be avoided. Finally, since polyunsaturated fats reduce the absorption of saturated ones from the gastrointestinal tract, whenever saturated fats are eaten, polyunsaturated fats should be eaten at the same time.

Vitamins. The body needs vitamins in small quantities to function properly. Since vitamins cannot be formed in the body, they must be supplied through food. Each vitamin has a specific action, and its deficiency gives rise to specific diseases. A discussion of all the various vitamins is beyond the scope of this book.

Cyanocobalamin (vitamin B_{12}) is essential for maintaining healthy nerve cells. A deficiency of this vitamin results in pernicious anemia, various neurological manifestations, and confusion. Patients who have gastric surgery are particularly at risk of developing vitamin B_{12} deficiency, and supplements should be prescribed, usually for life.

Ascorbic acid (vitamin C) is important for the formation of most tissues of the body, and a patient with a vitamin C deficiency may have delayed healing of wounds and hemorrhages. Late and severe cases of deficiency are known as scurvy. The role of vitamin C in protecting against the common cold is still controversial. Vitamin C deficiency is particularly likely to occur in patients whose diet is poor in fresh vegetables and fruit, and vitamin C is easily destroyed by cooking and reheating.

Although vitamin deficiencies may occur in elderly patients, there is no evidence that vitamins should be taken routinely if a person is healthy and eating a well-balanced diet. On the other hand, there is evidence of vitamin toxicity when large quantities of vitamins (particularly vitamins A and D) are taken unnecessarily.

The prevalence of malnutrition and vitamin deficiency in institutionalized or hospitalized patients has been well documented. In one Veterans Administration hospital, protein-calorie malnutrition was diagnosed in approximately two thirds of patients over 65 years of age; with younger patients protein-calorie malnutrition occurred in fewer than one third of the patients. It also was observed that infections and anemia were more common in the malnourished, geriatric patient. Further, malnutrition on admission indicated a significant increase of morbidity and mortality during the hospital stay.

Dietary fiber. The term "dietary fiber" refers to any substance of plant origin that is neither digested nor absorbed in the gastrointestinal tract. Examples are cellulose contained in fresh and dried fruits and vegetables and bran.

Dietary fiber remains in the lumen of the gastrointestinal tract and increases the bulk of the stools. Moreover, since fiber has water-attracting and -retaining properties, the consistency of the stools is rather soft and constipation is unlikely to develop. This is particularly important with patients with Alzheimer's disease, who are likely to become constipated or to ignore the call to defecate and consequently may become fecally inpacted and incontinent of feces.

SUMMARY

Currently there is no evidence that either nutritional deficiencies or nutritional intoxication are responsible for Alzheimer's disease.

The nutritional requirements of elderly people are to a great extent unknown. Because patients with Alzheimer's disease are very much at risk of becoming malnourished and dehydrated, caregivers must be alert to the patient's nutritional requirements and intake and ensure that his nutritional state is adequately monitored.

BIBLIOGRAPHY

Abalan F: Alzheimer's disease and malnutrition: a new etiological hypothesis, Med Hypotheses 15(4):385-393, 1984.

Birchall JD and Chappell JS: Aluminum, chemical physiology, and Alzheimer's disease, Lancet 2(8618):1008-1010, 1988.

Kamath SK: Taste acuity and aging, Am J Clin Nutr 36:766-775, 1982.

Lestou AP and Price LS: Health, aging and nutrition, Clin Geriatr Med 3:253-260, 1987.

Munro HN: Nutrient needs and nutritional status in relation to aging, Drug Nutr Interact 4(1-2):55-74, 1985.

Bernard MA, Jacobs DO, and Rombeau JL, editors: Nutritional and metabolic support of hospitalized patients, Philadelphia, 1986, WB Saunders Co.

Shore D and Wyatt RJ: Aluminum and Alzheimer's disease, J Nerv Ment Dis 171(9):553-558, 1983.

Singh S, Mulley GP, and Losowsky MS: Why are Alzheimer patients thin? Age and Ageing 17:21-28, 1988.

Yokel RA et al: Aluminum intoxication and the victim of Alzheimer's disease: similarities and differences, Neurotoxicology 9(3):429-442, 1988.

8

Sex and Alzheimer's disease

J. Turnbull

Before specifically discussing sex and sexuality in patients with Alzheimer's disease, it is appropriate to look at the broader aspects of this issue in regard to the elderly.

Every day in the United States, 5,000 people become 60 years of age. Many people, including elderly people, believe that individuals of that age have no interest in sex. However, interviews with elderly individuals at Duke University and other institutions have produced an overwhelming body of data indicating that people do not cease being sexual at 60, 70, 80, or 90 years of age. One man who was 103 years old was still sexually active! The problem is one of attitude.

Love and sex in individuals over 60 years of age are seen by most of the rest of the population as one of two extremes: cute and sweet, or dirty and depraved. The latter picture, of course, is more destructive. This is illustrated by mother-in-law jokes or cards that can be bought in stores depicting ugly, old women pursuing male athletes. A language full of words such as "old goats" and "lechers" symbolizes the attitude of a society that is obsessed with youth and beauty and that does not see the elderly as attractive, let alone sexual.

Despite this prevailing attitude, the sexual relationship between a man and a woman remains a central part of the being. In youth, sex and love often are separate and distinct, but as people age, the two aspects become inseparable. If for some reason a partner ceases to be sexual, the other feels rejected and unloved and worries about his or her attractiveness.

Individuals with Alzheimer's disease, as a result of the confusion and memory loss, may cease to be sexual. Because of this their partners should be more assertive in initiating and maintaining the sexual aspect of the relationship, for both their sakes. In many patients, particularly in the course of Alzheimer's disease, sexual drives may be absent.

One reason for the negativity towards sex in the elderly is the prevalence of preconceived ideas about being old. For example, some years ago I was lecturing to a high school biology class, and as part of my preparation for the class, I gave the students, a list of adjectives. There were 10 complimentary adjectives and 10 negative adjectives. I asked the students to choose 5 from the 20 that best described people over 60 years of age. These are the adjectives they chose: boring, sick, deaf, stupid, and querulous. Then I asked the class, "How many of you know someone over 60 who does not qualify," everyone except one student raised a hand. I said to this young woman, "How come you didn't hold your hand up?" She said, "I don't know anyone over 60; all four of my grandparents are dead." I said, "Where did you get your ideas from?" and she said, "television."

People's attitudes are shaped in part by the fact that they are afraid of getting old themselves. They are afraid of wearing out. They are afraid that they are going to be diminished physically, and most of all they are terrified of dying. As Woody Allen once put it, "I do not wish to achieve immortality through my work. I wish to achieve it through not dying."

Also, Western civilization tends to glorify beauty and youth. For instance, a woman over 60 years of age has never been a centerfold for Playboy Magazine, supposedly the paradigm of American female sexuality.

There are two forms of aging, biological and sociological, or sociogenic. Sociological aging derives mainly from society's attitudes toward the elderly. These attitudes vary considerably from culture to culture, as can be seen from the following true story. In China, where medical resources are limited, an 83-year-old man was brought to the local hospital in one of the rural areas. He had been badly burned in a house fire; burns covered 47% of his body, and his legs were burned almost beyond recognition. The surgeon in the emergency room said to the people who had brought the man in, "There is nothing we can do for him." The villagers replied, "You don't understand sir, you have to do something. We have brought this man 25 miles on a stretcher. We hand carried him because he is the most important man in our village." "Why is he the most important man?" "Because he is the founder of 'Former Poor Peasants,' and he was on the Long March with Mao Tse-Tung, and you have to save his life, because our village needs him." The surgeon said, "But if we take off his legs, he will probably die on the operating table." The man from the village said, "Is your vanity so great that you are afraid to lose a patient on the operating table? We need him." How many American residents of a neighborhood would take the same attitude toward one of their elderly neighbors had been badly burned? Probably not very many. How many people would come to the emergency room and demand that the man be kept alive? That is the difference in attitude.

Biological changes in sexual response and activity are also important. In women, for example, the most significant biological change that affects sexuality is menopause. Menopause does not mean that a woman's sexuality has come to an end, but some American women believe that this is so. Why? Because their husbands believe it. This is particularly true in two cultures that I have worked with in the past, the Native American culture and the Mexican-American culture. The men say to their wives, "Your reproductive days are over, you cease to be a sexual being, I'm no longer interested in you, move into the other room." After menopause, the estrogen levels are lowered, which may cause drying of the vagina. When the vagina is dry, sex sometimes is painful and this may lead to an aversion. Physicians, nurses, nursing assistants, and others who work with the elderly should inquire about this condition, because it can easily be corrected.

As a woman ages, she is more likely to develop any one of a number of illnesses that may interfere with her ability to be sexual. The impact of some of these illnesses upon sexual functioning is described later.

For men, the biology of aging is more serious as it affects sex. A man's refractory period, the time between erections, begins to lengthen at about 20 years of age, but it does not cause problems until about age 50. The refractory period becomes more prolonged each year that passes if the man does not remain very active sexually. As a rule, a young man of 17 years of age can have sexual intercourse and then have another erection 20 or 30 minutes later (in some young men it takes only 5 minutes). At age 70, the refractory period may be as long as 2 days. Many men are very worried about this, as they begin to recognize a diminution in their sexual performances.

Most men over 50 years of age have at least one incident of impotence. It may happen when the man is very tired, when he has been drinking too much, or when he is ill. After one episode of impotence, many men begin to worry about it happening again, and this worry may itself cause additional episodes, triggering a vicious cycle called performance sexuality.

Other biological changes also affect men: The penis may not be as firm as previously during erections, and the strength of orgasms or climax is lessened. Men often need reassurance about these changes, which are normal.

One important difference between men and women as they age is the life expectancy. In early adulthood the ratios of men to women are almost equal; in the United States, after 60 years of age there are three women for every man. After 70 years of age there are seven to eight women for every man. This means that if a woman loses her partner after the age of 60, the likelihood of her finding another man is very slim. A man, on the other hand, after the age of 60 may find himself actively pursued for the first time in his life. He may not know how to handle this situation, and the ensuing anxiety may cause impotence.

A number of medical conditions can affect sexuality in patients who have Alzheimer's disease.

One such condition is heart disease. In general, heart disease does not mean that a person's sex life should come to an end. It is often stated, "If you can climb two flights of stairs, 10 steps each, without getting out of breath and without getting angina, you can engage in sexual intercourse." It is less stressful to engage in sexual intercourse than to have an angry argument. However, many drugs given to patients with heart disease affect erections in men and lubrication in women.

Diabetes is another illness that often affects patients later in life. In women it causes difficulties in lubrication of the vagina and in achieving excitement. In men it causes impotence.

Arthritis causes sexual difficulties not only because of the pain in movement, but because arthritic joints may prevent movements essential in sexual intercourse. Patients should exercise and keep their joints mobile. Before engaging in sexual intercourse, they should nap or rest, lie down for a while, or perhaps take a warm bath. They also may want to take their medication just before engaging in sexual intercourse. The unaffected partner should be told in advance that an exclamation of pain should not cause him or her to cease activity.

Other tips cover position and timing: The so-called spoon position or vaginal rear entry position is more comfortable for the patient with arthritis than the traditional missionary position. Sexual intercourse in the morning, after the person has rested all night, may also be preferable to activity at night, when the person is tired and in pain. Some women avoid early morning sexual activity because of the ensuing pelvic congestion and resultant discomfort during the day. This can be avoided by ensuring that orgasm occurs.

Stress incontinence may be a problem, particularly for women if the incontinence occurs during intercourse. A woman with this type of problem should be advised to empty her bladder before intercourse. Kegel exercises may also be helpful. These are exercises in which the woman tightens the perineal muscles by squeezing as if stopping the flow of urine halfway through. The patient should perform these exercises approximately 150 times a day. They are very simple and can be performed while engaged in other activities such as standing by the sink or riding in an automobile. Kegel exercises also increase the strength of orgasm in women. Some cases of stress incontinence may require surgery.

Men may be troubled by prostatitis. With this condition the prostate is inflamed, and the patient has painful ejaculation that may be bloody. This disorder must be treated with appropriate antibiotics.

Many older men suffer from benign prostatic hypertrophy, or enlargement of the prostate. Others develop cancer of the prostate. In either case the prostate gland must be removed surgically. Such operations often but not always cause changes in penile erection. In some cases impotence results, particularly when nerves have been cut. Some men develop retrograde ejaculation, meaning that at orgasm the semen enters the bladder rather than the penis.

Self-stimulation of the genitals is common in both men and women. It may serve to release sexual tension in the absence of a partner. When it is done publicly, however, it elicits anxiety and disgust in others, and it may be seen as threatening to staff members and other patients. In institutions masturbation in public is often an expression of boredom, lack of stimulation, and most of all, the absence of being touched. One method used to reduce its incidence is to ensure that patients receive regular body massages of the shoulders and back, often with skin lotions after bathing. Also, patients should be told that such behavior is more suited to a private setting; they should not be disciplined by being placed in restraints, as sometimes is done.

IMPROVING THE SEXUAL RELATIONSHIP IN THE ELDERLY
Attitude

Unfortunately, many elderly individuals' attitude toward themselves directly reflects society's attitude toward them. Their attitude about sex is fixed but not unchangeable; it is shaped by their raising and reinforced by their experience. If a patient has had a poor sexual relationship for most of his life, then it is going to be very difficult to change later in life. If he has had a good sexual relationship, it is likely to continue.

Drugs

Many drugs have an effect on sexuality; antihypertensive drugs have been mentioned. Drugs that affect the mind (psychoactive drugs), particularly neuroleptic drugs such as thioridazine (Mellaril) and haloperidol (Haldol) reduce desire, excitement, and orgasm. Antidepressants and sedatives also affect sexual performance. Patients should be advised not to display their medications like trophies; the partner, seeing several bottles of pills, is unlikely to find this sexually arousing.

Affairs

The spouse of a patient with Alzheimer's disease, particularly one in the later stages, may become involved in an extramarital relationship. Because the partner is unable to satisfy the sexual needs, the spouse may look elsewhere. The caregiver should neither condemn nor condone such behavior but rather should attempt to listen and understand that sexual needs continue even in the absence of a willing partner.

Privacy

Living with children or in an institution makes it difficult to be private. Privacy in a nursing home is difficult to achieve, particularly if a person's spouse spends a great deal of time in bed, if someone else is in the same room, if there is no lock on the door, and if the nurses are always in and out. Some nursing homes have a privacy suite, which is set up something like a motel room, so that people can have some privacy.

Photographs

Many older individuals keep photographs of their loved ones in the bedroom after the death of a partner or a divorce. Beginning a new relationship with all the relatives looking down from the wall may prove to be sexually inhibiting.

SUMMARY

Patients with Alzheimer's disease and their spouses can engage in sex until the patient has reached the end-stage of the disease. As with any other illness, patients should be encouraged to maintain the sexual relationship for as long as possible.

BIBLIOGRAPHY

Breicher EM: Love, sex and aging, Consumers Union, New York, 1984.

Butler RH and Lewis MI: Sex after sixty: a guide for men and women in their later years, New York, 1976, Harper & Row, Publishers, Inc.

Dunn ME: Psychological perspectives of sex and aging. Am J Cardiol 61(16):24H-26H, 1988.

Ehrlich G et al: Roundtable: helping arthritics deal with sexual difficulties, Med Aspect Hum Sex 17:52-66, 1983.

Hsueh WA: Sexual dysfunction with aging and systemic hypertension, Am J Cardiol 61(16):18H-23H, 1988.

Kazdin AE: Behavior modification in applied settings, ed 3, Homewood, Ill, 1984, The Dorsey Press.

Pfeiffer E, Vervoedt A, and Wang H: The natural history of sexual behavior in aged men and women, Arch Gen Psychiatr 19:753-758, 1968.

Starr BD: Sexuality and aging, Ann Rev Gerontol Geriatr 5:97-126, 1985.

9

Ethical issues in the care of the patient with Alzheimer's disease

S. Turnbull

CASE STUDIES

1. Matthew J. is 62 years old and has a wife and three grown children. Two years ago he was diagnosed as having stage 1 Alzheimer's disease and was informed of this diagnosis. He has just recovered from a mild heart attack, and his cardiologist has told him that he requires cardiac bypass surgery if he is to live. He has refused the surgery, stating, "There is no point in living." The consulting psychiatrist confirms that Mr. J. is clinically depressed in addition to having Alzheimer's disease, and the psychiatrist believes that Mr. J. cannot make a rational decision.

2. Shirley W. is a 74-year-old patient with Alzheimer's disease who lives in a nursing home. Over the past few months she has become increasingly difficult to spoon-feed, spitting and pushing the spoon away and refusing to eat. When admitted to the home, while coherent and clear-minded, she had asserted that she did not want her life prolonged by artificial means. The physician orders feeding by nasogastric tube, which Mrs. W. frequently pulls out. In response to complaints from the nursing staff, the physician prescribes tranquilizers for Mrs. W. to make her "more manageable."

3. Dave S. is taken to his family doctor by his wife and grown daughter to find out why he has become so irritable. He admits to angry outbursts for no apparent reason and says that he has trouble remembering and is finding it increasingly difficult to add and subtract. After extensive testing, the diagnosis is confirmed: Mr. S. has Alzheimer's disease. The doctor tells him and gives him a broad outline of what he can expect. Mr. S. takes the news calmly, then states that under no circumstances does he want his wife or daughter informed.

4. Martha J.'s children have complained to the nursing home administrator that on their last three weekly visits, they have found Martha in her room, dressed only in her slip. The children have protested that "the nurses aren't even bothering to tidy her up." Actually Martha recently had become combative each time a staff member had tried to make her dress for social activities. The nursing staff, with feeling of ambivalence, had decided to honor Martha's apparent wish not to dress as long as she was in her room.

Caregivers charged with responsibility for a patient with Alzheimer's disease continually wrestle with ethical issues. Simple day-to-day care demands a repeated confrontation with these dilemnas. Dealing with the complex problem of the demented elderly arouses intense discomfort in the caretaker, especially when an ethical issue underlying the care emerges. Yet there are no simple answers, no agreed-upon formulas that can ensure that the rights of the demented elderly are maintained and that the conscience of the caretaker remains clear. Ultimately, every caregiver has a professional obligation to carefully analyze the ethical principles that must guide care, to explore her own moral boundaries, and to be aware of the need for respectful consideration of the impact of ethical issues on the quality of staff interaction and relationships.

ETHICAL PRINCIPLES GOVERNING CARE

Moral standards and the nature of moral decision making are the concerns of ethics, and ethical reflection is an obligation of the caregiver. Moral obligations sometimes are thought of as rules and indeed may be codified into law, but ethical practice goes far beyond what can be reduced to rules.

Certain values are basic to any ethical system. These are moral obligations in the sense that, without them, no community or cooperative activity could exist. These central values include truthfulness, fairness, and a respect for life. Besides these values, there are others, such as not inflicting harm of suffering. Caregivers often must make decisions in the face of conflicting values; telling the truth about the diagnosis of Alzheimer's disease may in itself cause suffering. Rules alone are not enough. Caregivers must thoughtfully consider whether actions and policies are consistent with moral principles and rules. Care of the patient with Alzheimer's disease presents many complex challenges to these moral principles, and the "good" choice is seldom obvious. But the caregiver is obligated to consider these issues carefully and to use them to frame moral choices to guide their behavior.

Three ethical principles are commonly applied to the dilemnas in patient care:

1. The principle of beneficence—that caregivers ought to produce good, preserve life, and prevent harm and suffering
2. The principle of respect for persons—that the autonomy and dignity of individuals should be preserved and promoted.
3. The principle of equity—that the benefits and burdens of care be fairly and equitably distributed among individuals.

PSYCHOLOGICAL REACTIONS OF THE CAREGIVER

The elderly demented patient, seemingly bereft of relationship and cognition, is often described by family and friends as "no longer here." In this sense the caregiver in the institution may have an advantage in that, not having known the "former self," she may find it easier than family or friends to see the patient as a full person, albeit one who is difficult, unpredictable, and complex. The family, on the other hand, grieves for the loss of the person they once knew and loved.

Caregivers themselves often experience powerful emotional reactions that profoundly influence their ethical decisions. Besides confronting their own mortality, they may see the frailties of the elderly demented as intimations of their own future losses, mental as well as physical. If the patient does not have a strong sense of individuality, a sense that depends largely on his ability to relate, the caregiver may project certain attributes onto him—often those of the caregiver's own parents—and respond to the patient accordingly. Many of the ethical dilemmas that caregivers face place them squarely in the center of a double-bind situation, where any action taken evokes guilt. For example, on the issue of forced feeding, caregivers experience conflicting demands—to preserve life (by techniques such as nasogastric tubes that may inflict additional suffering on the patient) and to respect patient's wishes (although refusal of food will shorten life). This double bind may increase the caregiver's sense of guilt or helplessness and impede ethical choices.

Little is known of the psychological mechanisms that caregivers use to manage their own feelings in these difficult situations. Undoubtedly many flee, choosing instead work that is less emotionally demanding.

Still others distance themselves emotionally from the patient, becoming less sensitive to his feelings and needs and eventually reducing their perception of him to that of "a thing. . . . handled routinely and mechanically, not nursed with tenderness and understanding." (Norberg and Norberg, 1980).

OBLIGATION TO PRESERVE LIFE AND PREVENT SUFFERING

The rigid stereotyping of professional roles, such as the physician's and the nurse's, may curtail the possibilities for successful management. Although current therapeutic measures cannot cure Alzheimer's disease, they can improve functioning and quality of life. Team efforts to resolve problems such as urinary incontinence and nocturnal agitation, for example, are often successful. Optimum care requires the involvement and collaboration of family members, friends, and caregivers alike. The question of what and how much life support should be given is a troublesome one, since loss of intellect often is deemed loss of humanness. Undoubtedly, the minimum ethical requirement is that the extent and irreversibility of the loss of cognitive function be established and that the patient be kept clean, adequately hydrated and nourished, and as free of pain and discomfort as possible. The ethical code embodied in criminal law prohibits positive euthanasia, the performance of a lethal act, even if motivated by a compassionate desire to prevent suffering. On the other hand, negative euthanasia, the decision to withhold treatment, and let nature take its course, is more generally accepted. Criteria for decision making are not well-defined, creating ethical dilemmas for conscientious caregivers. The patient's wishes, expressed while still competent, if known, should be considered. Ethical caregivers must

walk a tightrope between resisting premature requests from weary relatives or staff to stop all life prolonging efforts up to the last. . . . situations in which health professionals are uncertain about what is best should be resolved in favor of extending life where possible. This should apply when friends or relatives strongly urge it. They will have to live with these decisions, in a way that health professionals do not, after the death of their loved ones. (Dyck, 1984)

At the same time, patients have the right to refuse life-extending treatment, and incompetence does not diminish that right. When a patient, family, and caregiver cannot agree that the time has come, decisions must be left to the courts.

OBLIGATION TO RESPECT THE PATIENT

Institutionalization inevitably brings the patient into contact with paternalism. In a setting where most or all aspects of the patient's life are regulated by the staff, his individuality is invariably sacrificed to some extent. No longer able to select what to eat or wear or when to sleep, patients often respond with either belligerence or psychological withdrawal and a steadily increasing dependence. However, research indicates that the degree of dementia improves, or at least progresses less rapidly, when patients stay active and are allowed some role in decision making about even minor aspects of their environment. The issue of competence to decide is obviously a matter of degree. Some patients are competent to make all decisions, some most decisions, some only a few, and others virtually none. Individualized, case-by-case assessments that are repeated periodically can limit the overzealous application of paternalism. Obviously such assessments require considerable effort and reduce bureaucratic efficiency.

In general, individuals are presumed to be capable of discerning their own best interest and pursuing it. Seen as autonomous and competent, a normal person has the legal and moral right to choose and to refuse. However, it is just this right to make reasonable choices that is the major issue in progressive Alzheimer's disease. What degree of autonomy can be left to the patient? And who is to decide, if not the patient? By its very nature, paternalism (limitation of patients' freedom and authority by the "wise and loving father") exists to do good—to protect the patient from the dangers of his own freedom, such as the freedom to starve to death. Much of the health care function is inherently paternalistic, so paternalism probably cannot be totally avoided. However, effort should be made to keep it within proper bounds.

The right to decide is most controversial when it involves the refusal of treatment, particularly treatment that would extend life. Recent ethical debates and court decisions have done much to clarify the patient's rights and the caregiver's obligations in decisions involving patients who are still competent. It is clear that the patient should not be forced to undergo treatment that is against his wishes, even if the treatment is for his own good. Although the caregiver has an ethical duty not to force treatment against a patient's wishes, she has the additional obligations of helping to educate the patient and helping him to work through the reasons for refusal. Two criteria have been identified as morally justified for refusing treatment—if the treatment is useless, or if it involves a grave burden for the patient or another.

But who should decide for the incompetent patient, and what criteria should be used? These questions are surrounded by much greater controversy. The concept of substituted judgment is increasingly being recognized by some states and validated by the courts in cases in which patients had expressed their wishes concerning care while they were still competent so that those wishes could be carried out even if they lapsed into incompetence, perhaps with the appointment of a guardian to ensure that their wishes were expressed. If the patient, while competent, does not express an intent (or if a patient has never been competent), other issues arise. Generally, when the care of an incompetent patient without a guardian is debated, the courts must decide in favor of what they deem to be the best interest of the patient. However, the extent to which family members rather that the courts should have the right to decide among the reasonable courses of action available is unclear. Veatch and others have argued for a "limited familial autonomy," wherein the family is given responsiblity for carrying the patient's or family's beliefs and values into the decision, with the caregiver seeking court intervention if the family is felt to be unreasonable and exploitative.

OBLIGATION TO GIVE EQUITABLE TREATMENT

The principle of equitable treatment provides for impartiality and prevents discrimination. It ensures that the patient's rights to adequate treatment for the preservation of life or prevention of suffering are in no way diminished simply because the patient has special characteristics, such as being elderly (or demented). Too often the right to impartial treatment is overlooked or ignored in patients with Alzheimer's disease. When cognitive decline prevents conventional types of interaction between the caregiver and the patient, the patient often is viewed as an undesirable patient. Yet "undesirable" is not valid ethical grounds for disenfranchising a patient from the normal standard of care. Three of the numerous ways in which differential treatment can be seen involve disclosure of the diagnosis, different management of medical problems, and the use of restraints.

Disclosure of Diagnosis

In the early stages of Alzheimer's disease, the patient can understand the diagnosis and prognosis. But should he be apprised of these facts at this time? Informing a patient of a diagnosis of Alzheimer's disease presents vexing issues. Under the principle of autonomy, the patient is seen as having a moral right to know. Adherence to the principle of beneficience, on the other hand, may lead to a decision to withhold this information if it is felt that it would be detrimental to the particular patient at that time. Although no studies have yet assessed the actual impact of being told, a study by Erde, Nadal, and Scholl suggests that an overwhelming majority of individuals (92%) indicated they would want to be informed of the diagnosis. Reasons commonly given included being able to plan for financial and personal care (94%), wanting to seek a second opinion (62%), and wanting to settle family matters (36%).

Those wanting to know the diagnosis were even more likely to want their spouse told (89%) if for some reason the information was withheld from them, and they also were more likely to state that not being told would make them angry (71%). The ethical caregiver balances the burden of being the bearer of bad tidings with a sensitivity to the patient's and family's needs, for spaced presentation of small "parcels" of information, for support and information at times when they request it and are able to accept and process it, and for help in coping with the signs and symptoms of the disease and in preparing for its progression.

Management of Medical Problems

The first duty of patient care, and the least controversial, clearly is a duty to provide care. Yet studies repeatedly have found that the institutionalized and the demented elderly seldom receive the aggressive medical care provided to patients who are more independent. Obviously, there is an ethical obligation to apply considerable effort, knowledge and skills in reaching a diagnosis of Alzheimer's disease, particularly in searching for other hopefully reversible causes of dementia. Likewise, the obligation to evaluate and treat fevers and physical illness is not diminished by the patient's age or mental state.

Restraint

The unpredictable behavior with Alzheimer's disease is often disturbing to caregivers. Disruptive behavior, "unprovoked" assaults, and combativeness are not uncommon. If such behavior is bothersome rather than likely to injure the patient or others, restraint is seen as unethical. Allowing the patient to stay in his robe, for example, may eliminate his resistance and prevent an assault. Unfortunately, physical or chemical restraints often are used to manage bothersome behavior, resulting in increased health risks from immobility, not to mention overmedication and drug reactions and interactions. What are the patient's rights in such a situation? An ethical decision would demand the use of the least restraint possible to ensure safety, not staff convenience.

BROADER ETHICAL ISSUES

Numerous ethical issues surround the difficult dilemmas of Alzheimer's disease. For example, what special protections are needed in research on Alzheimer's disease? This is a disease that requires experimentation on people, since no animal models have been identified. What is the ethical responsibility of the health care professional for assuring that research into the cause and amelioration of this frightening disease receive high priority? What are the implications for public policy, and what choices should be made about the allocation of scarce health care resources for this special group?

Underlying all these considerations, and central to the resolution of the ethical dilemmas presented by this disease, is a need for a unifying goal that can guide the care of the patient with Alzheimer's disease. Faced with a patient's inevitable disintegration into a disabling dependence that is devoid of meaningful relationship, the caregiver must ask herself, "What must be my goals?" I suggest two: to help the family and friends celebrate the individual personhood that once was the patient's and to grieve its passing, and to help make each moment for the patient "as gentle, as content, and as kindly as it can be." (Howell, 1984)

BIBLIOGRAPHY

Campion EW: Ethical issues in the care of the patient involved in Alzheimer's disease research. In Melnick VL and Dubler ND, editors: Alzheimer's dementia: dilemmas in clinical research , Clifton, NJ, 1985, Humana Press.

Cassell CK and Jameton AL: Dementia in the elderly: an analysis of medical responsibility, Ann Intern Med 94:802-807, 1981.

Dyck AJ: Ethical aspects of care for the dying incompetent, J Am Geriatr Soc 32(9):661-664, 1984.

Erde EL, Nadal EC, and Scholl TO: On truth telling and the diagnosis of Alzheimer's disease, J Fam Pract 26(4):401-406, 1988.

Goldman R: Ethical confrontations in the incapacitated aged, J Am Geriatr Soc 29(6):241-245, 1981.

Hermann HT: Ethical dilemmas intrinsic to the care of the elderly demented patient, J Am Geriatr Soc 32(9):655-656, 1984.

Howell M: Caretaker's views on responsiblity for the care of the demented elderly, J Am Geriatr Soc 32(9):657-660, 1984.

Norberg A, Norberg B, and Bexell G: Ethical problems in feeding patients with advanced dementia, Br Med J 281:847-848, 1980.

Veatch RM: An ethical framework for terminal care decisions: a new classification of patients, J Am Geriatr Soc 32(9):665-669, 1984.

POTENTIAL COMPLICATIONS

10

Urinary incontinence

R. Hamdy

Urinary incontinence is the inappropriate and involuntary passage of urine. Its exact prevalence is difficult to establish, because it can occur in varying degrees and in many instances the patient may deny having the problem. This is particularly the case with patients with Alzheimer's disease.

RELUCTANCE TO ADMIT INCONTINENCE

In the early stages of Alzheimer's disease, when the patient still has insight into his condition, he may try to conceal his incontinence so as not to draw the attention of his coinhabitants and social contacts. The patient knows he has a problem with his mental state, which he already may find difficult to cope with and to hide from his immediate social contacts, and rather than admitting his problem of urinary incontinence and seeking medical advice, he often resorts to concealing it. He may hide soiled clothes or wear towels in his underwear. Not infrequently the patient feels ashamed of having lost control over his bodily functions, in addition to difficulties with his mental state, and he may be embarrassed to mention it. Finally, he may be afraid that he will be forced to accept institutional care and to give up his possessions and independence. In fact, urinary incontinence often is the factor that convinces relatives and caregivers that institutionalization is necessary.

URINARY INCONTINENCE AND ALZHEIMER'S DISEASE

Frequently, the urinary incontinence seen in the early stages of Alzheimer's disease is not related to the disease itself but is caused by an unrelated condition that often can be easily treated. This is discussed later in this chapter. Unfortunately, the patient often feels that the urinary incontinence represents yet another step in his gradual and relentless deterioration and loss of control over his mind and now over his sphincters. This usually leads to profound depression punctuated by bouts of irritability when the patient becomes angry with himself and fails to understand what is happening to him.

In late stages of Alzheimer's disease, urinary incontinence often is the result of the underlying condition and the global reduction in the number of cerebral cortical neurons (nerve cells). Because of this reduction in neurons, no inhibitory impulses are sent out from the micturition center in the brain to the urinary bladder (this is explained further later). Alternatively, the patient may voluntarily empty his bladder in inappropriate places because he is totally unaware of his environment and completely disoriented. When the patient reaches that stage, he may also become incontinent of feces and his mobility is greatly reduced.

DISCUSSING INCONTINENCE WITH THE PATIENT

The treating physician and other caregivers must be alert to the problem of urinary incontinence and be prepared to discuss it openly with the patient before its impact undermines the patient's self-confidence, worsens his general condition, and disrupts his precarious equilibrium with his environment. The caregivers must stress that urinary incontinence is not necessarily related to Alzheimer's disease and that it may be possible to correct it. Unfortunately, a conspiracy of silence often develops when the patient, the relatives, and care-givers know that the patient is incontinent and yet pretend not to have noticed it.

It also is remarkable how often the patient's relatives try to conceal the problem, and when questioned they may deny that their relative is incontinent until the situation becomes intolerable, in which case often little can be done apart from seeking institutional care. This is unfortunate, because even in late cases, a reversible cause for urinary incontinence sometimes can be found and successfully treated.

COMMON TYPES OF URINARY INCONTINENCE

A number of classifications for urinary incontinence have been put forward. However, patients often have more than one type simultaneously. The various types are not mutually exclusive, but often potentiate each other.

Stress Incontinence

Stress incontinence characteristically occurs when a patient stands up, coughs, laughs, or sneezes. The patient usually is dry in between these episodes and at night. Stress incontinence is caused by weakness of the urinary sphincter and/or perineal muscles, which cannot prevent small quantities of urine from being passed when the intraabdominal pressure is suddenly increased (as occurs during sneezing, laughing, and coughing).

Stress incontinence also may result from anatomical changes interfering with the urethrovesical angle (the angle between the urinary bladder and urethra). In women, this may be a result of several pregnancies and childbirth or surgical interventions. In addition, estrogen deficiency in postmenopausal women often leads to urethral inflammation, which is associated with senile vaginitis that may further aggravate stress incontinence. In these instances the diagnosis can be suspected by the appearance of the vagina and can be confirmed by microscopic examination of a mucosal smear.

Stress incontinence often is aggravated by diseases that cause muscle weakness or interfere with the patient's mobility, such as Parkinson's disease, strokes, or osteoarthritis. In these instances the patient may have to strain or heave himself as he struggles to get up from his chair. This straining increases the intraabdominal pressure, which is transmitted to the urinary bladder. If this pressure exceeds that of the urinary sphincters, urinary incontinence results. A similar situation may arise when a patient tries to get up from a very low chair. Stress incontinence is more common in women and usually responds well to pelvic floor and perineal muscle exercises (Kegel exercises).

Urge Incontinence (Detrusor Instability)

Urge incontinence results when uninhibited contractions of the detrusor muscle (the muscle layer lining the urinary bladder) are strong enough to overcome the pressure of the internal urethral sphincter. This type of urinary incontinence is also known as unstable bladder, spastic bladder, or uninhibited bladder, and it is the most common type of urinary incontinence in old age. It is characterized by the almost continuous passage of small quantities of urine, with the patient being wet most of the time, day and night, in a manner similar to newborn infants. The patient may feel the desire to micturate but is unable to postpone it.

In late stages of Alzheimer's disease, detrusor instability is caused by decreased cortical inhibition, because the number or integrity of the neurons in the micturition center of the brain is affected, in which case uninhibited contractions of the bladder occur before the bladder reaches its full capacity. Stress incontinence often potentiates detrusor instability.

Detrusor instability also may be caused by local or pelvic processes, including inflammation, infection, prostatic hypertrophy, neoplasms, fecal impaction, uterine or bladder prolapse, and foreign bodies such as calculi in the urinary bladder.

When urinary tract infections are responsible for this type of urinary incontinence, the incontinence usually is associated with a certain amount of dysuria (pain or burning sensation while passing urine). It must be emphasized, however, that although acute bladder infection often is responsible for incontinence, chronic infection does not always lead to urinary incontinence.

Overflow Incontinence

As with other types of urinary incontinence, overflow incontinence occurs when the pressure inside the bladder exceeds the pressure of the internal urinary sphincter. Unlike all other causes of urinary incontinence, however, overflow incontinence is caused by an actual obstruction to the flow of urine through the urethra. As a result of this obstruction, urine is retained in the bladder, which progressively increases in size. The pressure in the bladder also increases until it exceeds the pressure obstructing the flow of urine, at which point urine is discharged from the bladder until the pressure in the bladder falls below that of the obstructing lesion. Characteristically, patients with overflow incontinence have grossly distended bladders that can be palpated clinically, and the urine flow rate is significantly reduced, often amounting to no more than a dribble.

One of the main problems with overflow incontinence is incomplete emptying of the bladder. A residual volume of urine frequently is present even at the end of a bout of incontinence (this is why the bladder is palpable). This residual urine invites bladder infections, which may spread to the kidneys via the ureters.

One of the most common causes of obstruction to the flow of urine in men is prostatic hypertrophy. However, many other causes may be responsible for urinary obstruction and overflow incontinence, including fecal impaction, pelvic tumors, urethral stricture, bladder neoplasms and calculi and, in women, also uterine or bladder prolapse. The obstructing lesion may distort the urethra enough to cause an angulation of the urethra and to obstruct the flow of urine, thus interfering with micturition.

Often when these patients try to micturate but cannot, they strain and increase the intraabdominal pressure which is transmitted not only to the intravesical pressure, but also to the base of the bladder and the structures surrounding the urethra. As a result of this increased pressure, the angulation of the urethra becomes more pronounced and further increases the obstruction and difficulty in initiating micturition.

There is another problem: As the intraabdominal pressure increases while straining, the venous return from the abdomen to the heart is reduced; this causes pelvic congestion and may further increase the volume of the obstructing lesion or the already distended prostate and further interfere with the initiation of micturition. The solution to this problem is simple and consists of not straining and taking deep breaths to decrease the pressure in the thoracic cavity and increase the flow of blood from the abdomen and pelvic cavity to the heart. This will reduce the intraabdominal and intrapelvic congestion (including that of the pelvic structures and urethra) thus reducing the obstruction to the flow of urine and allowing micturition to take place.

Drug-Induced Urinary Retention and Overflow Incontinence

Occasionally, overflow incontinence may be precipitated by sedatives and tranquilizers that have anticholinergic properties.

Not infrequently, drugs that cause constipation (narcotic, antidiarrheal, and antidepressant drugs) may lead to fecal impaction. In severe cases the fecal masses in the rectum may distort the urethra, alter the angle between the urethra and urinary bladder, and cause urine retention and eventually overflow incontinence.

Antidiarrheal agents often are abused by elderly patients and their caregivers. Initially these compounds may be taken because of a bout of diarrhea or loose movements. If the patient continues to take them after the diarrhea has been controlled, he may become constipated, and in severe cases fecal masses, may become impacted in the rectum and later in the descending colon. Water is gradually absorbed from these fecal masses which become hardened (fecoliths). These in turn irritate the mucosal lining of the descending colon and rectum and increase mucus production. This may be interpreted by the patient as another bout of diarrhea, and he may take more constipating agents. As time goes by, the fecal masses may reach the proximal part of the descending colon, where the fecal matter is semisolid. At this stage the fecal material bypasses the fecoliths and may reach the rectum. The patient may not be able to control its evacuation and may think he has another bout of diarrhea and take more constipating agents, thus completing the vicious cycle and worsening his condition.

Functional Incontinence

Functional incontinence is caused by factors outside the urinary bladder and its nervous connections, which are all intact. The patient is incontinent of urine because he is unable to postpone the act of micturition until a suitable place for voiding is reached. In other words, the patient feels the desire to micturate, may start taking appropriate steps to go to the toilet, but does not have enough time to reach the toilet before micturition takes place. Stress incontinence often potentiates this type of urinary incontinence.

Curtailed patient mobility

Not infrequently, functional incontinence may result when a patient becomes less mobile. For instance, patients with severe osteoarthritis, Parkinson's disease, strokes, or any other condition that limits their physical capabilities may suffer from functional incontinence. In these instances it is often useful to advise patients to anticipate when the urinary bladder is likely to be filled and to attempt to void it at regular intervals of 2 to 3 or 4 hours rather than waiting for the urge to micturate to be felt. If the patient has Alzheimer's disease and cannot remember to empty his bladder at regular intervals, the caregiver may have to remind him. Alternatively, an alarm clock may be used to remind the patient to go to the toilet at certain intervals. In institutions a bladder-emptying schedule could be devised.

Inability to find the way to the toilet

Patients with Alzheimer's disease are prone to developing functional incontinence because they cannot find their way to the toilet. They may become incontinent because the toilet is at quite a distance from their bedroom or sitting area. The maximum distance between toilet and room or sitting area should be about 30 yards.

Similarly, if the way to the toilet is not clearly illuminated or if there are many obstacles on the way to the toilet, the patient may not be able to reach the toilet before his bladder empties. It must be remembered also that patients with Alzheimer's disease are likely to forget the way to the toilet. Thus it is important to make sure that the patient has easy access to the toilet, that he knows the way there, and that the way is well marked with signs. This is particularly important in institutions where a patient may wake up at night wanting to void his bladder but is confused and cannot recognize the way to the toilet. This is especially likely to occur during the first few days after admission to a nursing home or other similar institution.

Physical restraints

Functional incontinence may result from the use of physical restraints, which frequently are used with patients who tend to wander, to fall repeatedly, or become aggressive. This is often the case with patients suffering from Alzheimer's disease. Even though patients in restraints feel the urge to micturate, they cannot free themselves to reach the toilet in time. The development of urinary incontinence in these patients often is a serious setback and may considerably increase their degree of frustration, irritability, and even violence. Such irritability and occasional violence will reassure the caregivers that using restraints was justified, and thus a vicious circle is triggered. Often the rate of deterioration is dramatically increased when sedatives may also be prescribed to "quieten" the patient. As a result, the patient's condition deteriorates rapidly, and the complications of being bedridden quickly set in. Nurses who use restraints must make sure that the patients empty their bladders at regular intervals and do not develop incontinence.

Inability to communicate

It also must be stressed that patients with anomia, aphasia, or other speech problems such as patients with Alzheimer's disease commonly have may not be able to notify the nurse appropriately of their desire to micturate. For this reason nurses dealing with such patients must develop a set of vocabulary signals or a ritual by which the patient notifies them of the desire to micturate. If this is not possible, regular toileting should be instituted. This will be discussed in greater detail in the Chapter 11.

Drug-induced functional urinary incontinence

Not infrequently functional incontinence is also precipitated by drugs. Loop diuretic drugs, (e.g., furosemide, bumetanide and ethacrynic acid), which suddenly increase the volume of urine by several fold, may lead to functional incontinence, especially if the patient does not expect this to happen after taking the tablets. By suddenly increasing the volume of the bladder, loop diuretic drugs also may lead to pelvic congestion. In some instances, particularly in men with prostatic hypertrophy, this may lead to obstruction of the flow of urine and eventually to overflow incontinence.

Characteristically, incontinence induced by loop diuretic drugs develops within a short time of taking these tablets. Thus patients taking these drugs and their relatives or the nursing staff should be warned of the sudden increase in the volume of urine likely to occur after this medication is taken, and it should be ensured that the patient is taken to the toilet at regular intervals after taking the tablets. Also, patients on loop diuretic drugs must be kept near a toilet, and they must know their way to the toilet. Similarly, these patients should not be encouraged to go on outings or for walks within a few hours of taking the diuretic drug without making sure that they have ready access to a toilet. It must be remembered that a bout of urinary incontinence, even an isolated one, could be so humiliating for the patient as to completely undermine his confidence and significantly accelerate the rate of decline.

Functional incontinence may occur during deep sleep and is not infrequently induced by potent hypnotic drugs, when the patient's sleep is so deep that even though impulses are reaching the micturition center in the brain, they do not elicit any response from the other areas of the brain. Since no inhibitory impulses reach the sacral plexus, micturition takes place.

INFORMATION FOR THE PHYSICIAN

Although the patient's physician must diagnose the cause of the urinary incontinence, often the physician's task can be eased considerably if the right information is provided. The caregiver therefore plays an active and important role in diagnosing and managing the patient with urinary incontinence.

Even before referring the patient to a physician, the caregiver should attempt to determine whether the patient has genuine urinary incontinence or whether the leakage of urine is accidental, such as having spilled from the urinal bottle or bedpan, as often happens with patients who are bedridden or with those who are confined to bed either by physical restraints or by cot-sides.

Characteristics of the Incontinence

Once it has been established that the patient is genuinely incontinent of urine, the caregiver should determine whether the incontinence is of recent onset or whether it has been a long-standing problem. The former has a better prognosis than the latter, since it is usually the result of some reversible disease.

Attempts then should be made to find out whether the patient is incontinent of urine all the time or whether this tends to occur at specific times of the day and whether it is related to taking certain drugs. Urinary incontinence that tends to be worse late in the morning could be caused by loop diuretic drugs taken earlier in the morning. On the other hand, incontinence that is worse at night could be related to hypnotic (sleeping) preparations, which may profoundly inhibit the higher cortical (brain) functions. This is particularly likely if the patient is taking large doses of hypnotic drugs or has had potent preparations prescribed for him.

As there are other instances of drug-induced urinary incontinence, it is essential to know all the medications the patient is taking and whether they were prescribed by a physician or bought over the counter. Certain drugs bought over the counter to assist in weight loss may contain diuretic preparations. Other drugs prescribed for allergies or the common cold induce sedation or produce anticholinergic side effects which may lead to urine retention and eventually to overflow incontinence.

It must be remembered that elderly patients and those with Alzheimer's disease may take or be given medications that have been prescribed for their friends, neighbors, or relatives. It is therefore essential to inquire in detail about **all** medications the patient is taking. The management of drug-induced urinary incontinence is fairly simple and consists of discontinuing the offending drug or perhaps substituting a less offensive one. It is nevertheless important to consult the patient's physician before discontinuing any prescribed medication, even if the drug is believed to be responsible for the urinary incontinence.

Next, the caregiver must discover whether the urinary incontinence is related to any of the patient's activities, such as standing up, coughing, laughing, or sneezing. If the patient tends to be incontinent while doing any of these activities, the diagnosis is probably stress incontinence. It has been mentioned already that this type of incontinence often responds to pelvic floor and perineal muscle exercise.

If the patient is not incontinent all the time, it helps to know how many times he needs to micturate, the amount passed, and if it is associated with any urgency, dysuria (pain on urination), scalding, difficulty in starting micturition, or dribbling. Whereas the presence of the two last symptoms suggests prostatic hypertrophy, the presence of the first three suggests a lower urinary tract infection. Finally, the patient should be asked whether he has any bladder sensation and whether he can voluntarily initiate and interrupt the act of micturition.

If the physician is given all this information before seeing the patient, the task of diagnosing the condition will be much easier and the diagnosis is more likely to be accurate.

Clinical Examination

Although the physician will want to perform a thorough clinical examination of the patient, it is important that he be told about the patient's mobility and physical capabilities. Patients with disorders that interfere with their mobility are more likely to have urinary incontinence (functional incontinence) than fully mobile patients. Obesity itself may be a factor aggravating urinary incontinence by weakening the pelvic floor muscles.

The physician's examination probably will include a rectal examination and, in women, a vaginal examination. Before making a diagnosis, the physician may also want to order certain laboratory tests and sometimes may refer the patient for urodynamic tests.

SUMMARY

In many instances urinary incontinence is not directly related to Alzheimer's disease, and it may stem from causes that can be treated successfully. It is important to adopt a positive attitude toward the management of urinary incontinence and to try to identify the underlying cause or precipitating factors. Even if the urinary incontinence cannot be corrected, a number of aids can be used to make the management of these patients easier and to lighten the burden on the caregivers. These aids are discussed in detail in the next chapter.

BIBLIOGRAPHY

Diokno AC, Wells TJ, and Brink CA: Urinary incontinence in elderly women: urodynamic evaluation, JAGS 35:940-946, 1988.

Hilton P: Urinary incontinence in women, Brit Med J 295:426-432, 1987.

Leach GE and Yip CM: Urological and urodynamic evaluation of the elderly population, Clin Geriatr Med 2(4):731-755, 1986.

Ouslander JG: Diagnostic evaluation of geriatric urinary incontinence, Clin Geriatr Med 2(4):715-730, 1986.

Resnick NM and Yalla SV: Management of urinary incontinence in the elderly, N Engl J Med 313(13):800-805, 1985.

Thomas TM et al: Prevalence of urinary incontinence, Brit Med J 281:1243-1245, 1980.

US Department of Health and Human Services: Urinary incontinence in adults, Consensus Development Conference Statement 7(5):1-11, National Institutes of Health, 1988.

Wells TJ, Brink CA, and Diokno AC: Urinary incontinence in elderly women: clinical findings, JAGS 35:933-939, 1987.

Williams ME and Pannill FC: Urinary incontinence in the elderly, Ann Intern Med 97:895-907, 1982.

11

Urinary incontinence: aids for management

M. Lancaster

Urinary incontinence is a disturbing problem for both the caregiver and patient. The patient may feel ashamed and embarrassed, especially if he needs assistance. The caregiver also may feel embarrassed if accidents occur in public places. The onset of incontinence is the "last straw" for many caregivers and often results in the patient's being placed in a long-term care facility. However, a number of products and aids can lessen the strain of incontinence on caregiver and patient, and finding the most appropriate form of management can enable the family to care for the patient at home for a longer period.

PATIENT MOBILITY

In many older people, especially those afflicted with dementia, impaired mobility and slow gait may be the causes of incontinence. Simply getting to the bathroom in time becomes a real challenge. The best management strategy is to make the toileting facility more readily accessible. Climbing stairs to reach an upstairs bathroom is inviting accidents for a person with impaired mobility or urge incontinence. The pathway to the toilet must be uncluttered, well marked, and well lit.

When getting to the bathroom constitutes a major problem, other methods are appropriate. If the patient is fairly mobile, portable commode chairs (potty chairs) can be rented or bought from medical equipment suppliers and placed by the bed and in the areas of the house where the person spends most of the day. There are several different types of commode chairs, and selection should be based on the individual needs of the patient and family. Some chairs have wheels, which allows easy movement of the chair around the house. Others have pans that slide underneath the seat and can be easily removed for cleaning. This type of chair can also be rolled directly over the existing toilet, thereby allowing the patient to use the bathroom facilities. Some commode chairs are extravagant, with upholstery and lids, and they double as regular cushioned chairs.

ELEVATED SEATS

Because older adults have less flexible hip and knee joints, going to the bathroom can be difficult and uncomfortable, since sitting down on the toilet and getting up from it are more difficult. Elevated seats that raise the height of the toilet seat are available and may help to make going to the bathroom easier and less painful. Additionally, handrails can be installed for added support in sitting down and getting up. If the patient has trouble maintaining an upright position or has a tendency to fall to the side, chair arms are available that can be placed around the toilet to provide an additional degree of safety.

URINALS/BEDPANS

For the immobile patient, hand-held urinals for both men and women are available at medical equipment supply stores and pharmacies. If this type of equipment cannot be located, a plastic bowl can be substituted for a woman's urinal, and a plastic milk jug can be adapted for men. Having a urinal nearby or easily accessible will help to eliminate much of the anxiety that accompanies incontinence.

The bedpan frequently is used for a patient who is confined to bed. Problems encountered with the bedpan include difficulty in voiding in the lying position and the possibility of spillage in the bed. This type of equipment is also awkward and uncomfortable if used for any length of time.

PATIENT CLOTHING

Manual dexterity may be impaired in the older person with dementia, so such processes as unzipping pants or removing pantyhose may interfere with the patient's ability to stay dry. There are many ways to be creative with clothing to make them easier to remove and thus to keep cleaner and dryer. Velcro strips can replace snaps, buttons, and zippers. Clothing with elastic waistbands can be quickly and easily removed. Undergarments are available with flap openings that eliminate the need to remove the undergarment. Wraparound skirts and dresses are convenient and inexpensive.

URINE COLLECTION DEVICES

If the patient's incontinence is not due to poor mobility, confusion, forgetfulness, or lack of manual dexterity but rather to some medical or physical problem, there are drainage and collection devices, as well as absorbant/protective devices, that can make management much easier. Drainage and collection devices are closed systems by which the patient's urine passes into either an internal or external catheter and flows through drainage tubing into a reservoir. Absorbant and protective products either directly contain the urine or serve as a barrier to protect clothing, bedding, and furniture.

Indwelling Catheters

Internal drainage/collection systems are commonly called indwelling catheters. These consist of a rubber tube (catheter) that is passed through the urethra into the bladder. The catheter remains in place and is connected to a much larger and longer piece of plastic drainage tube outside the body. The urine passes directly into the catheter and flows to the collection device. The indwelling catheter system generally is used only if other management products and plans have proven ineffective. Because this device is inside the bladder, it provides a direct route for bacteria to enter the body, and urinary tract infections are a common complication with this type of system. Because of this, sterile technique must be used in catheterizing a patient, and the tubing should not be disconnected. Indwelling catheters should be changed on a regular basis, and the area where the catheter enters the body should be cleaned daily with an antibacterial solution (such as betadine). The patient's urine should be observed for signs of infection, including cloudiness, mucus, or blood. The patient should be encouraged to drink plenty of fluids and should be monitored for other signs of infection: lower abdominal or back pain, fever, increasing restlessness, pulling at the catheter, increasing lethargy, or confusion.

External Catheters

The external catheter provides a safer alternative to the indwelling catheter. For men, the condom catheter is the most frequently used drainage and collection device. This is usually a thin latex condom that fits over the penis and connects to a drainage tube. The condom should have some sort of firmer molding at the connecting end to prevent the thin condom from being twisted and closing off the drainage of urine. An external catheter usually is held in place by an elastic adhesive strip that fits either between the penile skin and the condom or directly over the top of the condom. The adhesive strip must be wrapped snugly around the penis to hold the catheter securely in place. However, extreme care must be taken not to make the adhesive strip too tight, as this can result in impaired blood circulation to the penis. If swelling or a change in skin color is noted, the adhesive strip is probably too tight and should be removed immediately.

External catheters should be removed daily, the skin washed with warm, soapy water, rinsed thoroughly, and dried well before a clean catheter is applied. Some patients, regardless of proper hygiene, will develop skin irritation underneath the catheter. This can be healed quickly by discontinuing use of the external catheter for a few days while relying on another form of incontinence management.

A few external collection and drainage devices are available for women patients; however, the female anatomy poses difficulty in using these products successfully. The female incontinence system usually consists of a pliable, funnel-shaped device that fits over the vulva and is held in place by pressure, straps, or adhesive. Some of these also use an undergarment that is worn to hold the funnel in place. Much more work must be done in designing an external collection system for women that is easily applied, comfortable, and effective.

Drainage Bags

The drainage bags or reservoirs for both the indwelling and external devices come in two basic forms; a leg bag and a chair/bed bag. The leg bag is a much smaller unit that holds a smaller amount of urine. These bags are strapped to the leg, which allows the bag to be concealed underneath clothing and enables the patient to engage in social activity without embarrassment or the need to carry around the larger reservoir bag. Leg bags are ideal for short trips, parties, or shopping. If the bag needs to be emptied while the patient is away from home, the urine can easily be drained into any toilet.

The larger bedside or chair bag is used mainly when the patient is at home or away from toilet facilities for long periods. Because these bags hold larger amounts of urine, they require emptying much less frequently and are ideal for nighttime urine collection. The large bag usually is transparent (at least on one side), which allows the caregiver to monitor the characteristics of the patient's urine. They are also marked in graduated increments, which is useful for monitoring the patient's total urine output. Because any type of drainage and collection system works by gravity, the collection bag and tubing must always be lower than the level of the patient's bladder.

Absorbant Pads

Incontinence management products that work by absorbing urine come in many styles and shapes, may be washable or disposable, and have various names. These products have become extremely popular over the past few years and have been marketed extensively as "the answer" to adult incontinence problems. Although many of the products work in essentially the same manner, serious considerations are involved in choosing the appropriate product. The availability of laundering facilities, the cost of the various products, and the degree of absorbency should be considered. Disposable products have the advantages of being much simpler and less time consuming than nondisposables. However, their cost may be greater in the long run. Also, the degree of absorbency and the ease of use may vary greatly. If the patient voids large quantities of urine, the volume of urine that the product will effectively contain should be of primary concern. On the other hand, if the patient's problem is occasional dribbling, a pad that is more comfortable and less bulky may be considered. Regardless of the type chosen, absorbent products have made life much easier and more dignified for many older adults. Because most of these products can be concealed beneath clothing, the individual can return to a more active and social life-style.

Adult Diapers

One of the most readily recognized incontinence products is the adult diaper. Basically fashioned after the diapers used with infants, adult diapers are good for people who are incontinent of both bowel and bladder. This product usually comes in sizes (S, M, L) and is fastened with adhesive straps or pins. Adult diapers have come a long way in incorporating elastic legbands and waistbands (to help prevent leakage), disposability, and stay-dry liners. Also, this product can be used with both ambulatory and nonambulatory patients. Although one of the bulkiest absorbent products, adult diapers can be worn underneath loose outer clothing. They can also be easily applied to bedridden individuals. Most adult diapers have absorbent inner layers covered by a waterproof outer layer. Frequently the layer next to the perineal skin will pull the urine to the outer layers, thereby preventing moisture from remaining in constant contact with the skin.

Adult Briefs or Pants

Adult briefs or pants are similar to underwear but have a pocket into which a thick, absorbent pad can be placed. When soiled, the pad is removed and replaced with a clean, dry one. This product also has a waterproof covering that prevents soilage of clothing. Adult briefs generally come in sizes according to waist measurement, thereby producing a better fit. They can be pulled on with an elastic waistband or snapped on. The product is a little less bulky than the diaper and is more suitable for patients who are socially active.

Because the slip-in pad may not be as absorbent as the adult diaper, the brief works best with patients who void smaller amounts or have a dribbling problem. Newer adult briefs are made of a very light, stretchable material with a waterproof area surrounding the pad. These newer products have also incorporated the stay-dry lining next to the patient's skin, thereby reducing the incidence of perineal rashes and excoriation. Differing from the disposable diapers, many adult briefs can be washed and reused, with the pad being the only item requiring replacement.

Protective Pads

Protective pads come in both reusable (washable) and disposable forms. As mentioned earlier, the major use of this type of product is to protect linens or furniture from becoming soiled with urine or feces. Several different sizes are available, depending upon the size of the area to be protected. When used to protect bed linen, the pad should cover an area that stretches from approximately midback to midthigh and out to the sides of the bed. This will promote protection when the patient turns and moves around in the bed at nighttime. A much smaller area can be covered when the patient is sitting in a chair, since less movement takes place.

At a minimum the protective pads should have a thin layer of absorbent material backed by a waterproof cover. Because an underpad is much less absorbent than the adult diaper or brief, it may need to be used in conjunction with one of the other incontinence products. Caution and care must be used with the protective pads, since they frequently roll or wad up underneath the patient when he moves. This can result in undue pressure to certain areas of the body and can eventually lead to skin breakdown if the pressure is not relieved. The protective pad should be straightened and all wrinkles removed when the patient receives care.

SKIN CARE

Regardless of the type of product chosen to aid in the management of urinary incontinence, particular and regular attention must be paid to providing good hygiene and skin care. The pad/pant/diaper should be changed whenever saturated and the skin cleansed with warm soapy water, rinsed well, and thoroughly dried. Proper skin care can prevent irritation and excoriation of the perineum. This area of the body should be monitored for signs of rashs or irritation just as would be done with a baby. Many of the skin care products used to prevent and treat diaper rash in children are suitable for use with adults. If a rash or irritation persists, the physician should be consulted. Occasionally, patients are sensitive or allergic to materials used in the products, and a rash develops. If this occurs, another brand should be tried before giving up on incontinence aids.

INSURANCE COVERAGE

Many of these incontinence management products are not covered by health insurance policies, Medicare, or Medicaid. Insurance policies should be checked carefully before assuming that incontinence management is a covered service. Because using these products can be expensive, an adequate workup to rule out reversible causes of the incontinence is encouraged.

SUMMARY

Urinary incontinence is a treatable and manageable problem faced by millions of people. It need not control the life of the patient or the caregiver. When the physician, family, and nursing personnel work together, a successful and amenable management plan can be developed. This leads to fewer worries, eases the burden and embarrassment, and allows a more normal and enjoyable life for both patient and family.

BIBLIOGRAPHY

Brink C and Wells T: Environmental support for geriatric incontinence, Clin Geriatr Med 2(4):829-840, 1986.

Burgio KL and Burgio LD: Behavior therapies for urinary incontinence in the elderly, Clin Geriatr Med 2(4):809-828, 1986.

Diokno A et al: Prevalence of urinary incontinence and other urological symptoms in the noninstitutionalized elderly, Urol 136:1022-1025, 1986.

Hadley EC: Bladder training and related therapies for urinary incontinence in older people, JAMA 256(3):372-379, 1986.

Kunin CM, Chin QF, and Chambers S: Indwelling urinary catheters in the elderly: relation of "catheter life" to formation of encrustations in patients with and without blocked catheters, Am J Med 82:405-411, 1987.

Thompson RL et al: Catheter-associated bacteriuria: failure to reduce attack rates using periodic instillations of a disinfectant into urinary drainage systems, JAMA 351(6):747-751, 1984.

Warren JW: Catheters and catheter care, Clin Geriatr Med 2(4):857-871, 1986.

12

Terminal care of patients with Alzheimer's disease

L. Norman

The symptoms associated with the third stage of Alzheimer's disease are marked irritability, seizures, emotional blunting, bulimia, visual deficits, decreased appetite, and muscle rigidity. Usually the patient is bedridden. He may become helpless, emaciated, and unresponsive or may progress to a coma. Caregivers have to remember that different patients progress through the stages of the disease at different rates, and not every patient goes through all the stages of the disease. This makes prediction of the rate of deterioration very difficult.

In the terminal stage of the disease, the person may no longer be able to be cared for at home. Institutionalization usually is necessary to provide for the patient's physical needs. Placing a patient in a nursing home may be a particularly difficult decision for families. The situation may seem hopeless for them, and they realize that the disease is irreversible. However, confronting the reality that the patient is in the terminal phase of the disease can be viewed positively by the family. Institutionalization may indicate relief for the family caregiver. The course of the disease has been very long and progressive, and the family has experienced a great deal of pain and stress trying to cope with it and with the changes that have occurred in their own lives. Many times family members may be very ambivalent about their feelings. They recognize that they will be relieved from the stress of being primary caregivers, but they feel sad, helpless, and even guilty that their loved one has to be institutionalized and probably will not return home.

Nursing care of the patient in the terminal phase of Alzheimer's disease must be based on the patient's specific problems. Also, close observation and added direct care are important during the terminal phase of the illness. As the individual becomes less able to participate in the activities of daily living, total care must be provided by the nurse or by the family caregiver if the patient is kept at home at this time. The caregiver's primary responsibilities are to meet the individual's basic needs and to assist him to a peaceful death.

VISION

Because visual acuity is diminished in patients with Alzheimer's disease, communication by speech and touch during the terminal phase is very important. The caregiver must sit or stand very close to the patient if he is to identify the person and understand any verbal communication. The patient may be easily frightened by someone entering his room, because he may not be able to see well enough to recognize his visitor. Calmness is essential for the caregiver; a sedate approach and a gentle touch will be reassuring. Caregivers should identify themselves and their purpose before any activity begins.

The patient's room should be comfortably illuminated and without glare. A dim light could be harmful, because it may create shadows that could cause the patient to perceive illusions of particularly harmful situations.

SPEECH

As the disease progresses, patients lose their ability to speak distinctly. As their speech begins to fail, the caregiver must anticipate their needs. By anticipating their needs, the caregiver should help them express as much as they can and talk to them as though they can reply. Caregivers should avoid talking around or even over the prone body of the patient. An example of this is when two people are changing a bed, and one tells the patient that they are going to turn him after the process of turning has already begun. Communication with the patient should be purposeful, not a rote response to an action. The caregiver should speak clearly and directly to the patient.

SKIN

The skin needs specific care. Patients may become thin and wasted because they have difficulty eating enough to maintain adequate nutrition. Their skin will be loose, and they lack sufficient adipose tissue to protect the bony prominences such as the sacrum, heels, hips, shoulders, elbows, and back of head. These areas must be protected from skin breakdown. Bedridden patients must be positioned and turned at least every 2 hours to prevent pressure sores.

The increased restlessness of the terminal phase causes additional problems with skin breakdown. Because patients may bump into the side rails and injure their fragile skin, padding should be used on the side rails. In patients prone to seizures during this phase, the padded side rails also help protect against injury during a seizure.

MUSCULOSKELETAL SYSTEM

The muscles and supporting structures may atrophy, which decreases support to the joints. Care must be taken when turning and moving the patient to keep from pulling on a joint and possibly dislocating it.

Range of motion exercises are important during this time to maintain as much mobility as possible, since the patient's muscles may progressively become more rigid. Maintaining function is imperative and is further discussed in Chapter 19.

RESPIRATORY SYSTEM

Some patients in the very late stages of Alzheimer's disease become short of breath. The chest muscles lose their elasticity, and breathing becomes more difficult. Also, the patients may be apprehensive, and restlessness may be the first indication of apprehension. Elevating the head of the bed and the shoulders helps the patient breathe more easily by decreasing the pressure on the diaphram.

As the respiratory muscles become rigid, the movement of the chest and the diaphram decreases. Because of this the patient can take only shallow breaths, and he usually is inactive at this time. These problems cause a pooling of secretions in the lungs. Stiffness of the muscles of the throat and chest may cause the patient to lose the ability to successfully cough and clear the respiratory tract of secretions. In this case a bulb syringe may be used to clear the secretions. If the patient is in an institution, suctioning the oropharynx may prevent secretions from occluding the airways.

Because they are unable to clear the airways completely, patients with Alzheimer's disease are prone to developing pneumonia in the terminal phase. The pneumonia usually is treated with antibiotics, which may be given intravenously, intramuscularly, or orally. The intravenous and intramuscular routes are fraught with problems. The patient is usually very restless and confused. Having an intravenous line only adds to the confusion, and the patient's activity may dislodge the needle. The patient also is often so thin that the intramuscular route is likely to be very painful. Usually the antibiotics are given by mouth or by nasogastric tube. During the terminal phase of the disease, the patient may have several bouts of pneumonia, even with the most meticulous of care in turning, positioning, and suctioning.

NUTRITION

The patient in the late stages of the disease has trouble swallowing, and pureed foods and liquids must be used to prevent choking. Asepto syringes or a Breck feeder may be used. It is imperative to feed the patient slowly. Aspiration of the food can occur if the patient is fed too fast with one of the feeding devices.

A nasogastric tube may be inserted to provide nutrition when oral feeding methods are not successful. Various liquid tube feedings are available commercially that provide adequate calories, protein, carbohydrates, and vitamins. Trying to persuade the patient to eat sufficient amounts by spoon or feeding devices may exhaust the patient and be a very time-consuming task. When a nasogastric tube is used for feeding, checking for placement before each feeding is very important. The patient's activity level and confusion could lead to misplacement of the tube.

FAMILY SUPPORT

As the patient with Alzheimer's disease reaches the terminal phase of the illness, the family needs help dealing with their feelings. The family may have experienced the phases of grief over the diagnosis and progress of the disease. However, some family members may be confronting for the first time the fact that their loved one is not going to get better and is going to die. The family needs to be supported as they deal with their feelings, especially since family members may be at various stages in their acceptance and not understand each other. One member may be in the denial phase and another in the acceptance phase of the process.

Dr. Elizabeth Kubler-Ross described the phases of grief as denial, anger, bargaining, and acceptance. During the denial phase, the person denies that anything is wrong or different. The family may have accepted that the patient has Alzheimer's disease, yet is unwilling to accept that he is in the terminal phase. A family member may point out how the patient is responding one day, such as breathing better, and may react negatively when anyone, caregiver or other family members, tries to tell her that the patient is getting worse.

Anger is expressed in many ways. A family member may verbalize anger that God caused this disease, that others contributed to the disease, or that they somehow caused the disease to occur in the patient. The anger may be directed at other family members or caregivers, on the grounds that if they had cared for the patient better, he would not be in the terminal phase.

Bargaining may be within oneself or with God. The family member promises to do many things if the patient will just live. As this is not effective, acceptance usually occurs. People experiencing grief vacillate between the stages; one day they may feel as though they have accepted that their loved one is in the terminal phase, and the next day there may be denial or anger.

It also is very difficult for the family to make decisions on resuscitation or treatment of infections during the terminal phase of the illness. Discussing the patient's wishes early in the course of the disease can help during this time. If a patient has expressed his desires about resuscitation, prolonged tube feedings, or other heroic efforts, it is easier for the family members to feel at ease in making their decisions. The professional caregivers must be sensitive to the family's wishes during the terminal phase of the disease and assist them in their acceptance of the patient's disease and condition.

UNIT FOUR
POTENTIAL IMPACT

13
Family education

M. Lancaster

*The outstanding memory I have, is of being abandoned by the
institutions I had formerly had a great deal of respect for. I had no
information from the doctor or the nurse in his office. I
inadvertently heard of the Visiting Nurses from the alternate doctor
in the office. They saved what was left of my sanity by giving me
information, as well as, three days help a week. I was reassured
that I was 'doing it right.' However, by the time I received this kind
of help, I was seriously near the breaking point myself. I had also
had eye surgery during this period. The medical and nursing
profession seem to have an important gap in their education.
Emotional and informational support seems to me of equal
importance with medical help. I received absolutely no
informational support. I stumbled onto what I needed accidentally,
and who knows what support was available that I never did
hear of.*

Sommers T and Zarit S: Seriously near the breaking point, *Generations* 10:30, 1985.

A number of areas of information must be explored with family
members who are caring for someone with Alzheimer's disease. Also,
providing this information helps the caregivers feel more competent in their role. Each member of the health care team must take
it upon himself or herself to become involved in the educational
process and to lend knowledge, expertise, and support to the family
caregiver.

OBJECTIVES

To properly educate family members of patients with Alzheimer's
disease, health care professionals must keep in mind the overall

objectives of their educational efforts. These can be generalized into three main categories:

Information on the disease afflicting the patient

Information on day-to-day care and management of the patient

Information on community resources

Armed with this information, the family will have the sense of support it needs to continue as the primary caregiver.

As educators of families, health care professionals must be knowledgeable about the impact that round-the-clock caregiving can have on a family. Caregiving normally takes its toll first on the family's free time (leisure and recreation). As the disease progresses and the patient's difficulties increase, caregiving begins to interfere with homemaking and work outside the home. Isolation also occurs, shrinking the family's support system and adversely affecting life satisfaction. In addition, the patient may take out his own frustrations on the caregiver, making the task of caregiving more difficult and emotionally burdened. The presence of an impaired person can severely disrupt the normal functioning of a family.

BASELINE INFORMATION

To appropriately address the educational needs of family caregivers, the health care worker must gather baseline information about the family. This begins with an assessment of the family's emotional state. If the family is currently in a state of emotional crisis, the crisis must be resolved or diffused before information can be absorbed. Any other sources of stress that are impinging on the family (unresolved financial or legal matters) also must be handled. The family should be assessed as to its ability to adapt to the changing needs of the patient and other family members. If the family members have not been able to adapt their daily lives to meet changing roles and demands, they may be unable to use the information provided or to apply it to their own situation.

Family members must be able to understand the information they are given. Asking the family what they know about the disease is a useful tool in determining the educational level of the caregivers. It is also an excellent way to find out what misinformation and misconceptions the caregivers may have about the disease and its management. Many of the problems and crises that caregivers experience evolve from misinformation or lack of information. Finally, it is important to find out if the caregivers are ready and willing to learn. If denial of the disease still exists, they will not be ready to listen to what is said.

PLANNING

Following the baseline assessment, the family caregivers must be involved in developing a treatment and education plan. Many caregivers are overwhelmed and confused when they first seek help. Their involvement in developing the plan helps in setting realistic goals for themselves and the patient. The gathering of the baseline assessment and the development of the treatment plan will be educational in themselves for the caregivers.

During these first two stages (assessment and plan construction), the family is given small pieces of vital information. This information helps to keep the caregivers going until they can be involved in more in-depth learning.

ONGOING EDUCATION

Education of the family is the basis of day-to-day management of Alzheimer's disease. The family should be taught about the course of the disease, symptoms, treatment, and medical and nursing management. Since Alzheimer's disease has several stages, educational efforts should concentrate on the stage in which the specific individual exists. Information about late stages is not relevant for caregivers looking after a patient who has just began to develop symptoms. Other topics that will need to be addressed include associated behavioral problems and their management, information about the aging process, common family problems resulting from the stress of caregiving, and available community resources.

A critical issue is the health care worker's own limitations as an educator. Each person has an educational style, some of which are more effective than others. It takes time and practice to communicate effectively with people and to relay information. No one has all the answers. Health care professionals must admit to themselves and to the family that because of the nature of Alzheimer's disease, the solutions and management trials offered are not going to work in every case. There will be times when "I do not know, but I will try to find out" may be the best response. If this is the case, getting back to the family with an answer is particularly important in maintaining the ongoing relationship with the caregiver that is centered on trust and honesty.

CRISIS PREVENTION

Anticipatory education (information before the fact) is vital. It may help to alleviate unnecessary emotional conflict and strain if the family has an idea of what the future may hold. Most families function on a fairly even plateau. The mere presence of the patient adds stress to the family's functioning and reduces intrafamilial harmony. Since patients with Alzheimer's disease tend to deteriorate slowly, the family usually has time to adapt to the additional stress. But as time and the disease progress, each additional impairment that the patient develops adds to the overall strain on the family and further reduces the harmony between family members. This continues until at some point even a very minor additional stress (e.g., the patient loses the car keys) makes the situation intolerable and induces a crisis.

Through anticipatory guidance and education, the family can be assisted to delay or possibly avoid this spiraling crisis. Therefore, if it is noticed that a patient has new problems or difficulties or that his condition is changing, preparing the family, ever so gently, for what behavior may lie ahead and providing management strategies can help allay fear and anxiety.

An ongoing relationship with a health care worker offers the family a real sense of security. Caregivers need to feel that there is someone they can turn to with their questions and problems. Many times this will be a member of the nursing or social work staff. Most families tend to have the feeling of, "we don't want to bother the doctor with this trivial question," and they turn to someone else. Generally, the caregivers need the piece of information or answer to their questions quickly and waiting until the next appointment with the physician may be too late. The family should be encouraged to keep a notebook on hand for jotting down questions, incidents, and problems. The notebook can then be taken to the physician's office or to a support group meeting for review.

Education on behavior management of the patient is probably one of the most important and most difficult tasks, because behavior varies so greatly between patients. Frequently, well-meaning caregivers can evoke a more severe reaction from the patient through lack of information on how to deal with certain behavior.

CASE STUDY

Mrs. M. was diagnosed 4 years ago as suffering from Alzheimer's disease. She is living with her daughter and son-in-law. One Sunday morning, Mrs. M's daughter instructed her mother to get dressed for church. Mrs. M had always been able to manage dressing herself. Fifteen minutes before they were to leave, the daughter found Mrs. M. crying in her room; she said she didn't want to go to church. The daughter, feeling rushed, insisted that her mother get dressed and go with the family. The daughter threw three of Mrs. M.'s favorite dresses on the bed and told her mother to hurry. Moments later Mrs. M. began screaming and tearing at her clothes. The daughter, angry at her mother for being so slow and childish, took one of the dresses and began to help her mother get dressed. Mrs. M. immediately began to fight with her daughter.

In the above example, Mrs. M. had suddenly been faced with her inability to dress herself. If her daughter had been prepared for this event, both may have reacted differently. Instead of rushing her mother, who was already overstressed, the daughter could have simply asked her mother if she needed help. Additionally, by forcing a choice on her mother, (which dress to wear), the daughter had added to the stress. The whole situation may have originally stemmed from Mrs. M.'s inability to decide what to wear. To spare both Mrs. M. and her daughter the final confrontation, it might have been most effective to redirect Mrs. M.'s attention to some other task. Once her mother had calmed down, the daughter may have been able to help her mother dress. Through anticipatory education and helping family members analyze their own interactions with the patient, the family can be assisted to see that their behavior may be contributing to the patient's troublesome behaviors.

CORRECT BALANCE

Well-intentioned families can also effectively block the patient's competence and capabilities by expecting too little from him. Being too helpful can promote apathy, dependence, and deterioration in the patient. This can be seen not only in patients with dementia, but also in patients who have had a stroke and in others suffering from chronic conditions. For example, if the patient begins to have difficulty feeding himself, the loving family member may come in to help feed him. Yet, the patient needs to practice feeding himself. Adaptive devices are available to make eating easier, and the family must be helped to accept spilled food, soiled shirts, and providing the patient with "finger foods." The family may need guidance on ways to allow the patient maximum self-sufficiency yet offering just enough assistance to compensate for the patient's real limitations. A delicate balance must be achieved between overcompensation and undercompensation.

FORMAL VERSUS INFORMAL TEACHING

Education can be carried out both in a formal manner and in an informal one. Family meetings with staff members are good mechanisms for formal teaching. These meetings are a good way to identify the specific behavior that is most troublesome to the family, how they explain the behavior, what solutions they have tried, and the effectiveness of their solutions. Family meetings are also an opportune time to discuss more sensitive issues such as legal and financial matters, wills, burial arrangements, and what will be done in the event of cardiac arrest. These matters must be discussed, and the assistance of the whole health care team makes the discussion much easier.

Informal education can be carried out at the bedside, in the home, over the telephone, or walking down the street. Role modeling is an excellent way to provide this type of education. Having the staff members and family members working side by side, be it a public health nurse in the home or staff nurse in a nursing home, affords each the opportunity to learn from the other. It must be remembered that education is a two way process. The family may be able to provide information on the best way to gain the patient's cooperation, whereas nurses can teach the family how to incorporate exercise into daily activities. Generally, the family has taken care of the victim at home for quite some time and is quite knowledgeable about the disease and the management of the patient. Health care workers must be accepting of the family's knowledge and experience and apply this information to care planning. The family should be encouraged to contribute to care plans. Frequently they have already discovered a solution to a problem that may be perplexing to staff members. It must be remembered that the treatment and management of Alzheimer's disease is still in the early stages of research—much of which is accomplished through trial and error.

A critical area of education that must not be forgotten is continuing education about aging in general and other problems or diseases that the patient might have. The family will need instruction on how to assess the patient for acute problems such as infections, pain, or fractures. They must be taught that the cognitively impaired person may not be able to relate signs and symptoms of acute conditions and that continuing physical assessment is vital.

WRITTEN INFORMATION

Education may be accomplished through verbal interaction, that is, sitting down and talking and working at the bedside with one another. However, verbal information must be supplemented and reinforced with written information. Numerous pamphlets and books are available and should be provided to the family. These resources are another vehicle for presenting education and providing hands-on information that the family can take home. For the caregiver, written material such as pamphlets serve as a reminder of the information verbally presented and as a step-by-step guide.

Written information can be individualized to meet the patient's and family's needs by writing down specific instructions and information in the margins of pamphlets and books. Much of the initial verbal information and instruction that is given to families is lost, because they are overwhelmed by the diagnosis and their attention is not focused on learning. The pamphlets and books provided can be reviewed over and over again at home when the family is more attentive and the information can be absorbed at their own rate.

Education of the family goes beyond learning about the day-to-day management of the patient and the disease. It must also involve education on what can happen to the caregiver and other family members and on the impact of caregiving on their family roles. Family members are very interested in possible cures and are susceptible to the media and the coverage that "breakthroughs" and "cures" receive. Families must recognize that the media frequently sensationalize this type of information. The family must be informed that some people will take advantage of their desperate situation. It is vital to encourage the families to investigate these advertisements carefully and to discuss them with their physician. They should be aware of side effects that may result from experimental treatments and the quality of life issues involved in the treatments.

OVERINVOLVEMENT

Overinvolvement in the care of the patient commonly occurs in an effort to compensate for the loved one's disabilities and loss of role in the family. When involvement with the patient is carried to an exaggerated extent, the caregiver may sacrifice many aspects of her own personal health and welfare. This is the major reason the caregiver becomes known as the second victim of Alzheimer's disease. Overinvolvement can lead to emotional and physical breakdown of the caregivers. Helping families to be aware of this tragedy and to know that they must take care of themselves to continue their caregiving role is of grave importance. Becoming emotionally and physically drained through overinvolvement can actually hinder caregiving and interaction with other family members.

ANGER

Anger is a problem that can arise at any time. It can arise within any member of the family and can be expressed between family members. Anger can be present in grandchildren because the patient is taking Mom's time away from them. It can arise between siblings over management methods. There are many reasons for anger: feelings of burden, abandonment, and embarrassment. Often this anger is displaced onto the patient, staff, or other family members. Understanding that anger is an emotion that is commonly expressed under stress can help the family to feel normal. They must also be able to recognize the anger and deal with it. Encouraging the family to talk openly and to express these emotions helps them deal with their feelings.

GUILT

Guilt is another emotion that is likely to arise within the family. Through education about the disease, its progression, and the other areas previously discussed, the family can be assisted to recognize that guilt is a normal emotion and that they are doing the best job of caregiving they possibly can. Common sources of guilt such as institutionalization or a family member's belief that he contributed to the disease should be discussed with the family.

ROLE REVERSAL

Role reversal and changes in family roles are likely to occur. The caregivers need to understand that they may have to assume some of the roles of the individual who has the disease. To assume the patient's roles and place within the family can be a very difficult and emotionally laden task. Through education the family can be helped through these changes and instructed on ways to lessen the impact these changes will have on the patient and other members of the family.

SUPPORT

Education and support should not be separated. They reinforce one another, and education can be effectively delivered in support groups. Providing information alone, without supplying a feeling of support, is not nearly as successful. The family needs the support of others to be able to assimilate the information they have received and to put it into practice. This is discussed further in Chapter 16.

BIBLIOGRAPHY

Buckwalter KC, Abraham IL, and Neundorfer MM: Alzheimer's disease. Involving nursing in the development and implementation of health care for patients and families, Nurs Clin North Am 23(1):1-9, 1988.

Cohen P: A group approach for working with families of the elderly, Gerontologist 23(3):248-250, 1983.

Chenoweth B and Specner B: Dementia: the experience of family caregivers, Gerontologist 26(3):267-272, 1986.

George LK: The burden of caregiving: how much? what kinds? for whom? Advances in Research, 8(2):2, Duke University Center for the Study of Aging and Human Development, 1984.

Hepburn KW and Gates BA: Family caregivers for non-Alzheimer's dementia patients, Clin Geriatr Med 4(4):925-940, 1988.

Ory MG et al: Families, informal supports, and Alzheimer's disease. Current research and future agendas, Res Aging 7(4):623-644, 1985.

Powell L and Courtice K: Alzheimer's disease: a guide for families, Reading, Mass, 1986, Addison-Wesley Publishing Co, Inc.

Roberts BL and Algase DL: Victims of Alzheimer's disease and the environment, Nurs Clin North Am 23(1):83-93, 1988.

Simank M and Strickland K: Assisting families in coping with Alzheimer's disease and other related dementias with the establishment of a mutual support group, J Gerontol Soc Work 9(2):49-58, 1986.

Skurla E, Rogers JC, and Sunderland T: Direct assessment of activities of daily living in Alzheimer's disease. A controlled study, J Am Geriatr Soc 36(2):97-103, 1988.

Smith CW Jr: Management of Alzheimer's disease. A family affair, Postgrad Med 83(5):118-120, 125-127, 1988.

Somners T and Zarit S: Seriously near the breaking point, Generations 30-33, 1985.

Wiancko D, Crinklaw L, and Della Mora C: Nurses can learn from wives of impaired spouses, J Gerontol Nurs 12(11):28-33, 1986.

Winogrond I et al: The relationship of caregiver burden and morale to Alzheimer's disease patient function in a therapeutic setting, Gerontologist 27(3):336-339, 1987.

Zarit S, Todd P, amd Zarit J: Subjective burden of husbands and wives as caregivers: a longitudinal study, Gerontologist 26(3):260-266, 1986.

14

Stress in health care workers

J. Turnbull

Stress has been defined in a number of ways. Hans Selye, probably the most famous writer on the subject, referred to stress as a physiological state that results when an organism is influenced by a stressor. Stressors include both physical stimuli (e.g., noise, heat, cold, pain) and psychosocial stimuli (e.g., death of a relative, moving into a nursing home, changing jobs).

Human response to stressors is mediated (influenced for good or ill) by personality, coping skills, and awareness of what is happening, which is sometimes call insight. Thus the stress of the job of caring for a patient with Alzheimer's disease is influenced by a variety of factors. A caregiver's resistance to the stressors of the job depend on what is being played out in the theater of her life. Marital squabbles, problems with children, and deaths in the family all influence the caregiver's ability to do the task at hand.

The stressors in the daily care of the patient with Alzheimer's disease include, from the patients: uncooperativeness, incontinence, heavy lifting, aggressiveness, failure to communicate needs, death, wandering, insomnia, and mood swings.

Most stressful of all is the lack of a time frame in which to make plans. In most other instances there is a clear prognosis or course. In Alzheimer's disease this is lacking. A patient may live for 1 year or 20 after a diagnosis is made, this uncertainty is very stressful.

Worker burnout, which is the direct result of stress, is fairly common among people who care for patients with dementia. It is a process that consists of three stages.

The first stage involves an imbalance between the resources and the demands placed on the resources. In other words, be it the health care worker or the family, the demands placed on them exceed their ability to deliver.

For example, a mother of teenage children who are undergoing their own life crisis is suddenly faced with the fact that her own parent is now unable to undertake the simple tasks of living without assistance. This mother has to sacrifice her time with her children, whose surliness and uncooperativeness increase in proportion to the lack of attention from their mother, who is caring for grandmother. The caretaker (mother) is placed in the middle and experiences demands beyond her ability to meet.

In institutions a similar situation may arise when the nursing assistant finds herself on a particular day caring for a disproportionately large number of very demanding residents because a coworker has phoned in sick. If this situation is compounded by the nursing assistant herself feeling unwell, but also responsible enough to feel she must be at work, a crisis caused by stress is about to develop.

The second stage is the immediate short-term emotional response which is characterized by tenseness, anxiety, and feeling exhausted.

The third stage consists of a number of changes that the health caregiver or family member undergoes, such as: a tendency to treat the patient in a detached and mechanical fashion or a cynical preoccupation with having her own needs met.

It can immediately be seen that burnout is a transactional process. In other words, it is an interaction between many different things; job stress, the strain on the health care worker or family member, and the way the individual accommodates psychologically to the whole process. What happens is that a previously committed person disengages from her work and develops a series of signs and symptoms.

INSTITUTIONAL SETTINGS

In an institutional setting, the signs and symptoms include the following:

A high resistance to going to work every day with frequent tardiness or even absenteeism. The thought of going to work when getting up in the morning is simply overwhelming.

A sense of failure.

Anger and resentment, particularly toward supervisors, the institution itself, and unfortunately, sometimes toward residents.

These feelings are followed by: guilt and blame, discouragement and indifference, and social isolation and withdrawal, as well as negativism toward life in general.

Individuals who are burned out spend time watching the clock during the day and feel tremendously fatigued after work. They come home and are unable to engage with their own families in any meaningful way. Some individuals that I have treated for burnout who worked with patients with Alzheimer's disease simply went home to bed and lay down for several hours, refusing to get involved with the family, with the preparation of meals, or with the daily chores.

There is also a loss of positive feelings toward patients and a tendency to clump them all together. The caregiver is unable to concentrate or to listen to what the patient is trying to say. There is a feeling of immobilization, of being unable to do anything about the situation. The caregiver then becomes cynical and blames the patients, as if it were their own fault that they are in the institution. There is a tendency to go by the book, to follow instructions in a mechanical way and to do the very minimum.

Then begins a series of psychosomatic complaints, including insomnia, avoidance of discussing work with colleagues, and self-preoccupation. The caregivers develop frequent colds, viral infections, headaches, and upset stomachs. They become rigid in their thinking and resistant to change.

Some individuals even become paranoid about their coworkers and the administration. This is the stage in which individuals may use drugs and alcohol, begin to have marital and family conflicts, and show a heightened rate of absenteeism.

THE HOME

Many of the problems of the family member who is charged with caring for the patient with Alzheimer's disease are the same as those of the caregiver in an institution. The guilt and blame, discouragement and negativism may all be experienced. However, the family member does not go home at the end of the day; she is already at home. There is little respite except in sleep, and even that may be disturbed. Such family members begin to experience a breakdown of their coping skills and like institutional caregivers, they may become physically ill.

STRESS AND PERSONALITY

As indicated earlier, the way individuals respond to the stresses of the job depends on their own personality traits, what they want to do with their lives, and what sort of experience they have had, as well as the quality of their life outside work. Individuals who have what is called an external locus of control are more vulnerable to burnout than individuals who have an internal locus of control. Individuals who have an external locus of control project all problems onto the environment and see themselves as victims. This applies to their whole life. They are not self-motivated but require tremendous amounts of stroking to continue doing their job. Individuals who start out being extremely humanitarian tend to burnout in institutions such as nursing homes because they don't see their work resulting in changes for good.

On the other hand, individuals with an internal locus of control accept that they are masters of their own destiny and require much less in the way of positive feedback to feel good about themselves. The person with an internal locus of control feels much less stressed about caring for a patient with Alzheimer's disease than his counterpart with an external locus of control.

Patients with Alzheimer's disease are rarely, if ever, openly appreciative of the tremendous amount of work done for them by family members and institutional caregivers. If being thanked, praised, complimented, and rewarded in some way is of paramount importance to a caregiver's well-being, she will be sorely disappointed in caring for the patient with Alzheimer's disease.

It must be realized that worker burnout always affects patient care. It is well known in psychiatric hospitals, on inpatient units, that high rates of suicide attempts, high rates of elopements from the unit, high rates of depression and general misery in the patients occur when the staff members are demoralized. This in turn increases the degree of stress the staff feels, and a vicious cycle has begun. Attempts to improve staff morale can turn this situation around. The staff members begin to feel better, and patients begin to do better.

DEFINING THE JOB

What every health care worker in the field of caring for the demented patient wants most is to prevent the job from becoming an employment slum. Nursing homes traditionally have not been high-prestige work locations—little glamour is attached to such a job. In fact, sometimes relatives of residents are abusive and demanding to staff members who are working as hard as they can. This abuse reflects guilt and shame, but it is hard for staff members not to take it personally. It is therefore important for nursing homes to be able to attract people who are content to work with chronically ill individuals and who are not already burned out and cynical about their jobs.

Part of an employee's enjoyment of her job is the professional stroking she gets from colleagues and the fact that she likes the people she is around. The friendships that she makes at work can be one of the most sustaining support systems imaginable. Interestingly, the problems of "glamour" also apply to the family caregiver. Community support is much more likely to develop when a relative has had a stroke or heart attack or has developed some other physical ailment that does not affect the mind.

PREVENTIVE MEASURES

How can burnout be prevented in people who care for demented patients? There are two aspects of prevention, individual and organizational. Interventions to alleviate burnout include the following:

1. The reduction or elimination of excessive job demands. In other words, more must not be expected of people than they can reasonably do.
2. A change in personal goals and preferences to meet the reality of the situation.
3. An increase in the caregivers' resources for meeting the demands of the task.
4. The provision of coping substitutes for the withdrawal characteristics of burnout.

Burnout in an institution is a highly contagious disorder and requires tremendous efforts to reverse. Such efforts are often met with resistance by a pessimistic and thoroughly demoralized staff. In almost no other situation is the old adage "an ounce of prevention is worth a pound of cure" so appropriate.

One of the simplest solutions, of course, is to hire more staff. Clearly an overload of work is a common cause of burnout in many human service agencies. However, the tendency to always define the solution as more resources has some very serious flaws. Researchers have also suggested that tremendous changes in staff-patient ratios are necessary before any substantial change can occur if this is the only step taken. Burnout has many other causes such as role conflict, the ambiguity of the definition of work, lack of variety, lack of autonomy and control over one's work, and destructive norms. These have nothing to do with the number of people hired.

STAFF DEVELOPMENT

One of the first ways in which intervention is possible and necessary is in staff development, which seeks to do the following:

First, to reduce the demands that workers impose on themselves by encouraging them to adopt more realistic goals. Second, to encourage the people who work in an institution to adopt new goals that might provide alternative sources of gratification. Third, to help the workers develop new monitoring and feedback mechanisms sensitive to short-term gains. In other words, reporting regularly to someone who listens to what a person has been able to accomplish and getting some positive feedback for it. Staff development should also seek to provide frequent opportunity for inservice training designed to increase role effectiveness. It should attempt to teach staff members coping strategies such as time study and time management techniques.

In my work with patients, one thing that I had to learn early was to be pleased with relatively small gains. New staff members who come onboard frequently expect to be world-shakers and to make tremendous gains in patients very early in their careers. Caregivers working with the elderly, particularly those with Alzheimer's disease, don't make many gains. Caregivers must also learn to work with patients' relatives, so they can give some positive feedback. Inservice training provides opportunities for individuals to learn new techniques for working with problems with patients or to redefine old techniques.

WORK LOAD

Another way in which burnout can be prevented is to change job and role structures. This can be done by limiting the number of people for whom staff members are responsible at any one time. This is particularly important for settings in which caregivers work with groups of ill patients. For example, suppose a program has 12 patients and three staff members. The staff members can either share the responsibility for all 12, or they can each take responsibility for four. Researchers have found that overload is lessened, when responsibility is divided. Even though the patient-staff ratio is no different, there is less stress when the group is divided into three smaller groups, and the staff members are assigned to these. The staff members also feel a greater sense of personal responsibility and control when they are solely responsible for a smaller number of patients.

It is also important to carefully select the mix of patients assigned to staff members. In general, the most difficult patients should not be assigned to any one staff member. It is common for newly hired staff members to be given the most difficult patients of all, but patients who are physically and morally repugnant or who are resistant and abusive, severely withdrawn or very handicapped should not be assigned to new staff members who have had inadequate training.

TIME-OUT

Most jobs in the human service industry allow little opportunity for reflection and thought. Yet these are absolutely vital for effective coping. Time-outs, which allow staff members to escape temporarily from the demands of the role and to think uninterrupted about what they are doing, reduce overload and strain.

One way of ensuring that time-outs will be available is to use auxiliary workers such as volunteers or part-time people. Vacation time policies also can be used to provide relief. Sometimes employees have to be encouraged to take frequent vacations. The tendency to allow vacation time to accumulate and to regard this as some kind of status symbol should be discouraged. Flexibility has to be maximized, so that people who can work take vacations on short notice whenever they need to. I remember in my work at one mental hospital how one staff nurse boasted to me that in 3 years she had taken no vacation time and now had accumulated over 8 weeks. I felt like saying, "No wonder you're such a lousy nurse."

Another difficulty arises over the use of people who want to work part-time. My own belief is that part-time workers are extremely beneficial to an institution, but unfortunately most institutions are so inflexible that they do not provide the fringe benefits such as medical leave, medical coverage, and insurance to part-time workers.

ADMINISTRATIVE SUPPORT

Administrators of institutions also have to think about ways to make life more pleasant and work more enjoyable for their staff members. One such approach is career ladders. Lack of career ladders has been identified as a major source of dissatisfaction in people who are not professionally trained. Career stages do alleviate burnout by enhancing the practitioner's vicarious sense of competence.

Competence is one of the most important aspects leading to self-esteem on the job. Human service work is expected to be more than just a job. It is a calling in the truest sense of the word. A caregiver prepares to work on an Alzheimer's unit or in a nursing home in a way that a worker does not when he becomes a factory worker, bartender, or postal employee. The greater preparation is emotional as well as financial and intellectual. Yearly merit raises that are given automatically are not enough to reinforce a caregiver's confidence. A true career ladder requires advancement in the form of meaningful increases in responsibility, privileges, and status.

Administrators and managers must know how to do their jobs properly. They must make their goals clear, develop a strong, distinctive guiding philosophy, and make education and even research a major focus of the program in which they are involved. Most of all, they must reinforce the belief that the people who are working for them and with them are doing a good job. It seems hard for supervisors sometimes to say "thank you" or to acknowledge that their staff members are working hard in somewhat unusually trying circumstances.

LAST BUT NOT LEAST

Finally, some personal aspects must be kept in mind. The value of friends who sustain a caregiver outside the job is often underestimated. The caregiver's relationships with the key people in her life must be worked on and polished. Sometimes outside help may be necessary to get back on track. One of the most encouraging recent developments in the United States has been the emergence of the Alzheimer's disease support groups, which are discussed in Chapter 16.

BIBLIOGRAPHY

Given CW, Collins CE, and Given BA: Sources of stress among families caring for relatives with Alzheimer's disease, Nurs Clin North Am 23(1):69-82, 1988.
Lecso PA: Murder-suicide in Alzheimer's disease, J Am Geriatr Soc 37(2):167-168, 1989.
Selye H: Stress in health and disease, Sydney , Australia, 1976, Butterworth Publishers.
Tennant C, Langeluddecke P, and Byrne D: The concept of stress, Aust NZ J Psychiatry 19(2):113-118, 1985.

15

Abuse of the patient with Alzheimer's disease

K. Mathews

FAMILY VIOLENCE

Whether it be child, spouse, or elder abuse, family violence is an age-old problem. It has been a very private problem, one that no institution or provider has addressed until recently. The closeness of the family unit and the fear of punitive outside intervention has kept clinical observation at arm's length. Only when friends chance by and observe possible abuse, or when medical attention is sought in emergency rooms, or when someone in the family reports it, does family violence come to the attention of the authorities. Therefore, abuse of any type is difficult to discover, categorize, and/or understand. When dealing with the possible abuse of a patient with Alzheimer's disease, an examination of the literature shows that we know even less about it than elder abuse generally.

There is evidence in the literature, both ancient and modern, that violence has been part of the family for hundreds or even thousands of years. The Oedipus' murder of his father, Laius, and his marriage to his mother, Iocaste, form the basis of a Greek tragedy illustrating family violence. The account in Genesis of Cain killing Abel illustrates some of the family violence themes mentioned biblically. Research on the view of yesteryear's family being a harmonious, multigenerational unit relying on mutual generosity and sympathy and characterized by the veneration of elder's is largely a myth.

Still, family violence is not yet properly understood. A number of different theories have been advanced to explain different types of violence in different subgroups of the family. None as yet are entirely satisfactory explanations. There is a belief that family violence has a number of antecedents with many different triggering factors. And both victims and potential perpetrators of family violence in general and in Alzheimer's disease in particular share many of these common antecedents. Whether abuse occurs in patients with Alzheimer's disease or whether some protective mechanism exists in this subgroup remains to be elucidated. Almost no one willingly reports abuse of any kind in any age group, especially the perpetrator. Legislation in the last 20 years dealing with some aspects of family violence has possibly made both health providers and perpetrators more reluctant to report, further obscuring the issue.

Following is a brief summary of the state of knowledge of the major components of family violence, preparatory to a discussion of the Alzheimer's disease subgroup.

Child Abuse

This generation of scientific inquiry has recently "scientifically discovered" family violence in the form of child abuse. The landmark article by Dr. C. Henry Kempe in the Journal of the American Medical Association in 1963 raised the possibility that bruises he was seeing on pediatric patients might in fact be deliberate rather than accidental. There is now a strong body of medical literature concerning the reality of child abuse. Each state has allocated considerable resources to identify and treat child abuse. It is a condition that is diagnosed with great reluctance and that is occurring more often.

Many physicians find it difficult to report a case of suspected or actual child or elder abuse because of personal feelings, physician-patient confidentiality and, not in the least, failure to recognize the condition. Awareness and detection are essential in formulating a plan for treatment and prevention.

Spouse Abuse

Although literature is scarce, spouse abuse merits consideration because it is a major component of family violence. It was "discovered" in the 1970s, and attempts were made to facilitate diagnosis and treatment, but care of the battered spouse largely became the domain of community volunteer agencies. No body of law was to be found nor was any created to rescue battered spouses from their abusers. Law enforcement agencies increasingly found themselves involved but were largely ineffective in dealing with the problem unless a spouse filed charges or obtained a restraining order. Domestic violence has been shown consistently to be one of the most dangerous interventions police are called upon to settle. Spouse abuse occurs widely but currently has no vocal group to aid in treatment and prevention.

Elder Abuse

It should be observed that at some point, generally ascribed to be 65 years of age, spouse abuse can become elder abuse. In the late 1970s, it was "perceived" that this subset of the family was also prone to abuse. Studies of the elderly have since shown their susceptibility to violence, much as the rest of the family unit is susceptible. It is within this group of older persons that we find those who are at risk for Alzheimer's disease.

It is necessary to describe elder abuse more fully, since most patients with Alzheimer's disease are part of this family subset. Because there is almost no literature on abuse of the patient with Alzheimer's disease, inferences will be drawn from the elder abuse data and suggestions for future research will be made.

Although child abuse laws are on the books of all 50 states, the elder abuse laws, modeled after child abuse laws, are on the books of 43 states. These laws require mandatory reporting of suspected elder abuse, as with child abuse, with much the same penalties for failing to report. These penalties include possible jail terms and/or fines. It is expected that soon all states will have a similar statute on elder abuse.

In general, these statutes state that failure to report a suspected or actual occurrence of elder abuse is a misdemeanor subject to prosecution. With this legislative intent, it can be seen why there is reluctance on the part of the Alzheimer's disease support groups, families, and caregivers to seek medical attention; they fear that they will be accused of abuse.

What are the estimates of the prevalence of elder abuse, and how do these estimates compare with those of child abuse? From the child abuse literature, we know that at least 4,000 children will die annually as a result of child abuse; 200,000 children will be sexually exploited, and 200,000 to 300,000 children will be psychologically abused. Totaling all types of child abuse gives us an estimate of perhaps a million cases of abuse. Much less certainty exists in the elder abuse literature on its prevalence. Estimates based on several limited surveys suggest that 500,000 to 1 million people over 65 years of age may be abused in some fashion. This represents roughly 4% to 10% of the population of those over 65 years of age. Estimates of moderate and severe abuse range around 4%, with the upper limit of prevalence of all types of abuse being as high as 10%. Perhaps as many as one in every 25 elderly Americans (1.1 million) may be victims of such abuse. These figures are similar to the approximately 1 million cases of child abuse reported each year.

Definition

There is a problem with defining abuse. Physical abuse is a more obvious part of the definition, since there is objective evidence of bruising, burns, or fractures. Both in child abuse and elder abuse, the definition has been widened to include neglect and exploitation.

Several lists of definitions of elder abuse exist. Failure to agree on the definitions of elder abuse both in the state laws and in the scientific literature has contributed to the misunderstanding of the disorder and to the confusion in the prevalence rates. Those categories most commonly accepted are briefly summarized here in an attempt to explain the abuse potential in a patient with Alzheimer's disease. The categories are passive neglect, active neglect, financial abuse or financial exploitation, and psychological abuse (some authorities include medical abuse). Last on the list is physical and/or sexual abuse.

Passive neglect. Passive neglect may represent nothing more than unintentional forgetfulness by the caregiver. Elderly patients who have no transportation and who live in isolated circumstances often run out of essential heart or blood pressure medicine and then return to the physician's office some months later with high blood pressure or heart failure. When they do manage to get to the office, they sometimes have been charged $5 or $10 by a relative to bring them in for evaluation. Some of these patients have had to be hospitalized immediately for uncontrolled diabetes or some other potentially preventable condition.

I have visited homes that had nothing but sour milk or rotting cottage cheese in a little cooler (no refrigerator), because the family members were too lazy or uncaring to stop by and bring fresh food or to cook the elderly relative something edible. By the same token, she may have just given them a hard time for trying to force her to leave her home or for any number of other reasons. Thus no one wants to go by to see her and be "told off" again.

This behavior may also represent a well-intentioned caretaker who is unable to meet the needs of the elderly person. The caregiver may be physically but not mentally capable of meeting the abuse victim's needs and may simply ignore them.

Active neglect. Active neglect is the failure of the caregiver to intervene and resolve a significant need of the patient. Examples include failing to visit isolated elderly people and neglecting to bring them food or clothing or to provide heating in the winter despite the awareness of available resources. Active neglect, in contrast to the passive type, is associated with malicious intent on the part of the caregiver. The end result is often the same; the elderly person is taken to the hospital or to the physician. The results of both passive and active neglect could have been prevented, but the results of failing to take preventive action are the same.

Financial exploitation. Financial abuse or exploitation is another common cause of abuse. This commonly occurs when a relative or some close friend of the patient oversees the patient's financial resources. Caregivers may withhold money and necessary services to conserve the patient's money for their inheritance. It is doubtful that a patient with Alzheimer's disease would be able to report financial abuse or exploitation.

One particular case illustrates this dilemma. An elderly patient of mine who was the matriarch of the clan was nearing total dependence on family members. Her husband was dead, and she was the deed holder of considerable property, on which some of the children and grandchildren already lived.

The social interactions over the years had taken their toll. Some children were favored, and some were not. The group of children who had fallen out of favor had been trying over the past several years to get the will changed and the patient declared incompetent. At one point they secured a subpoena from the judge and had the sheriff's department take her to the physician's office for a determination of competency. Fortunately for the patient, the doctor thought she was still competent. Since then other family members had taken to staying with her around the clock to prevent this from happening again.

I became involved when they asked me, as their family physician, and another physician to certify her as competent. With this documentation she would be able to change the will and dispose of the estate during her lifetime. I understand that the will was changed according to her wishes. She subsequently became unable to oversee her affairs and may in fact be incompetent in the disposition of her own care. This is not an unusual case, and it appears to have a happy ending. Many times elderly people are swindled without their knowledge.

Another such case is illustrative. A 75 year-old gentleman recently came to see me accompanied by a neighbor. The chief complaint was that he had become so childlike that a stranger from Florida, who had moved into the area, secured his confidence and then bought his 10 acres of country real estate for almost 90% less than its market value. When the neighbor heard of the transaction, it was already to late to stop it. A lawyer had advised the neighbor that he needed three physician's statements certifying that the man was unaware of his loss. I presumed that this would in some way establish incompetency in an attempt to nullify the transaction, if in fact it was possible. Unfortunately, this occurs all too frequently in this day and age.

Psychological abuse. Psychological abuse occurs when the caregiver behaves in a way that restricts the patient's freedom or reduces his self-worth. The patient may be locked in a room and told not to come out until papers releasing money, stocks, or dividends are signed. Loss of privileges may be another form of abuse. There are many variations of psychological abuse, and it is likely to be both a serious and significant problem but vastly underreported.

A common form of psychological abuse consists of disparaging comments made directly to the older person or to others in their presence. Remarks such as, "You are so stupid," "How can you keep forgetting things?" or "Can't you take better care of yourself?" lead to loss of self-esteem and may even cause depression.

Physical and/or sexual abuse. Physical and/or sexual abuse is a very serious component of abuse of the elderly, because patients often cover up for the person who is abusing them. Observers may see a bruise, chafing marks, or a rope burn from being tied in the wheelchair or some other problem but may not recognize it as abuse. Fear of being taken from their home and fear of institutionalization are the major reasons patients cover up this abuse; they also may be further abused by the caregivers for telling the authorities.

One particularly common form of physical abuse is the use of restraints. Since patients with Alzheimer's disease are prone to wander and sometimes fall, caregivers devise means of restricting their mobility. Methods of restraint include tying the patient to the bed with sheets and placing them in Geri-chairs (lounge chairs with lap tables that can be screwed in place). While restraining a patient may be necessary for short periods of time, it becomes abusive when patients are left tied down for hours, unable to go to the bathroom, to scratch an itch, to relieve a painful area or even to roll over in bed. Sometimes the restraint itself increases the patient's irritability and agitation, which the caregivers may use as additional reasons to continue the use of restraints.

Psychotropic drugs to reduce the irritability and wandering behavior are often overused and may constitute a form of physical abuse. Indeed, some national organizations such as the American Psychiatric Association have felt compelled to produce written guidelines for the use of this medication to prevent abuse.

It is unknown whether patients with Alzheimer's disease, who are a subset of the elderly population, suffer more or less abuse than those without dementia or whether they are protected from abuse in some way because of their disease.

Risk factors of abuse. Victims of abuse are more frequently women than men. More than 55% of victims are 75 years of age or older. In approximately 75% of the cases, the victim lives with the relatives. Victims often have significant physical or mental impairment and are unable to meet their daily needs without assistance.

Dependence is another risk factor. Victims who have relatives dependent on their home, income, and transportation are more likely to be abused.

Dependency is such an important concern it should be examined more closely. Any older person may be injured and become dependent on a caregiver, and this dependency is extremely disruptive to the caregiver's family. Depending on the severity of the disability or disease process, family caregivers may spend their entire waking day baby-sitting the person. Caregivers lose sleep, jobs, vacations, financial resources, and so forth to maintain the disabled person.

A study in England of patients with dementia compiled the major reasons caregivers end up taking the elder to an institution. Table 1 describes the nature of and the tolerance for the dependant's behavior problems as identified by those caring for them before admission to the hospital or institution.

It can be immediately seen from this table that caregivers are very intolerant of patients who fail to sleep through the night but are extremely tolerant with problems of daily living.

Two conclusions are suggested by the table: First, as the patient's behavior becomes more difficult, the likelihood increases that he will be admitted to an institution. Second, the caregiver loses tolerance as the behavior becomes more difficult to handle. These disabilities increase the likelihood of abuse as the dependency on the caregiver increases. Are patients with Alzheimer's disease, with many of these impairments, as likely to be abused as are those without dementia? Research is needed to answer this question.

Caregivers may make several attempts to cope with their patients. Some caregivers are more resourceful than others and survive longer in their role. Those caregivers who decompensate may end up abusing the patients, placing them in a nursing home, or taking them to the hospital. What are some of the reasons caregivers become frustrated? What problems are more likely to cause abuse, institutionalization, or hospitalization?

Table 1 Tolerance of Care-givers to Various Behavioral Problems

Behavior Problem	Tolerance (%)
Sleep disturbance	16
Micturition in inappropriate places	17
Shouting	20
Inability to get off commode unaided	21
Inability to get on commode unaided	22
Night wandering	24
Daytime wandering	33
Inability to walk unaided	33
Inability to get out of bed unaided	35
Dangerous, irresponsible behavior	38
Incontinence of feces	43
Inability to get into bed unaided	40
Physically aggressive behavior	44
Inability to communicate	50
Personality conflicts	54
Inability to manage stairs unaided	60
Falls	62
Inability to eat unaided	67
Inability to dress unaided	77
Incontinence of urine	81
Inability to wash and/or shave unaided	93

Adapted from Sanford SR, Br Med J, 3:471, 1975.

Profiling the caregiver shows that a caregiver who abuses a patient is a relative in 86% of the cases. The son and the daughter are the most likely to be the cause of the abuse, but any live-in relative or friend can be an abuser. The caregivers generally are under stress from work, either from being unemployed, having too much work, or being dissatisfied with their job. In three fourths of the cases, the caregivers have problems with alcoholism or drug abuse or are in poor health.

Elder abuse and Alzheimer's disease

There are no studies yet specifically linking elder abuse with Alzheimer's disease. Likewise, no studies of Alzheimer's disease have yet to report any incidental findings of elder abuse. One such example of the absence of information is illustrated here.

The University of Michigan completed a study on the experiences of family caregivers coping with patients with Alzheimer's disease. This study selected 413 families at random from the mailing list of the Minnesota Chapter of the Alzheimer's Disease and Related Disorders Association (ADRDA) and sent them a questionnaire. The family was asked to describe their experiences with coping with the diagnosis, treatment, and care of the patient. The questionnaire did not ask specific questions about abuse.

The families' answers did not reveal a single response about any kind of abuse or the possibility of wanting to be abusive, although there were numerous statements summarizing the frustrations of caring for these patients. The study concluded simply that families of dementia patients do experience a great deal of emotional stress during the relative's illness.

The lack of data at this point makes it impossible to determine the extent of abuse of patients with Alzheimer's disease. It is possible to make some statements on the similarities in the two populations and to suggest some directions research might take to answer these questions.

The first similarity between elder abuse victims and patients with Alzheimer's is that of age. By age 85, "severe" dementia is present in more than 15% of that age-specific population. Age is also a prerequisite for elder abuse. The elder abuse victim tends to be 75 years of age or older. Thus there is virtual overlap between the population of older persons and persons at risk for Alzheimer's disease.

The second similarity in the two groups is the commonality of physical or mental impairment leading to disability. It already has been established that elderly people with physical or mental impairment are much more at risk for abuse. Does it follow that patients with Alzheimer's disease, with their progressive dementia, likewise have an increased risk for elder abuse?

A third similarity is dependency. There is dependency by the victim on the caregiver, and often a counterdependency by a caregiver on the victim. It is well understood that patients with Alzheimer's disease become progressively more dependent on their caregivers. This dementia, along with likely physical impairment that may occur in old age, can produce situations requiring total supervision of care for a prolonged period of time.

As noted previously, a significant case-control study mentioned dependency of the abuser on the abuse victim as a risk factor for elder abuse. Is this dependency process in elder abuse similar to or different from the dependency process in Alzheimer's disease? The case-control study questioned from its findings whether dependency of the victim was as important a risk of abuse as was the dependency of the abuser on the victim.

This finding may suggest that socio-economic levels of families with patients with Alzheimer's disease may play a role in determining the risk of abuse. That is, the fewer the resources of the caregiver, the more increased the dependency potential on the victim and thus the increased potential for abuse. Families of patients with Alzheimer's disease that have greater resources might be in a lower risk situation for abuse. This has yet to be investigated.

SUMMARY

A number of observations have been made on the populations at risk for elder abuse and Alzheimer's disease. Similarities in risk factors have been outlined for both groups. The size of the population at risk has been assessed and found to be large. Even though the information on elder abuse is limited, there is virtually no information on abuse of patients with Alzheimer's disease. Are there as yet unknown factors that limit abuse in Alzheimer's disease, or is the abuse as yet unreported? Does the double stigma of abusing a known patient with Alzheimer's disease who is frail and elderly drive the problem deeper into the closet?

Both groups of victims are vastly under recognized and thus under reported by medical providers. This is especially true when abuse is something other than physical or when the Alzheimer's disease is in its early stages. Is under reporting of abuse in all types of older persons due to an old family secrecy, the fear of public exposure and judicial punishment? Will laws on reporting abuse increase the prevalence of abuse and decrease the reporting of the disorder? Is the potential stigma of abusing a defenseless patient with Alzheimer's disease so great that no one is likely to report it if it occurs?

With so great a population of elderly people at risk for Alzheimer's disease, is it reasonable to expect abuse to occur in that population? If abuse truly does not exist in the Alzheimer's disease population, then researchers must determine the factors that reduce the possibility of abuse in this group. This knowledge could be used to reduce the prevalence of elder abuse and to prevent new cases from occurring.

Raising the index of suspicion in the medical provider community and in the public at large of the possibility of elder abuse is crucial to developing an understanding of this disease. Increased awareness could lead to early intervention and prevention. Elimination of existing abuse and prevention are the ultimate goals.

Should a Caregiver Report Abuse?

The laws in most states provide that if a caregiver *suspects* or *observes* abuse, she must report it to the State Department of Human Services. Abuse is generally defined as physical abuse, neglect, or exploitation. Failure to report such carries a penalty of fines and/or imprisonment.

These laws are very similar to the Child Abuse Protection Act. They also provide for anonymity for the reporter and immunity from prosecution should discovery occur. The Department of Human Services has a legal obligation to make a visit and determine two things: Is the alleged victim in imminent danger of death, and is he competent to refuse services if offered? Many times there is no imminent danger of death, but services are needed. Many times the client refuses the services.

The major difference between Child and Adult Protective Services is the ability of the child case worker to remove the child from the home without a court order. An adult may eventually be removed, but a court order is necessary if the removal is involuntary. This legal protection for the adult also makes it difficult to provide for the needs of the client. Even if the need is severe, the client must accept the services voluntarily or be competent to refuse them.

Prevention of Abuse

The goal of any responsible abuse program is to prevent it before it occurs. Treatment programs may aid victims but are often too late. Prevention remains the major goal of all providers.

What can be done? Unfortunately, specific prevention of elder abuse in any special population of the elderly is as yet unknown. Abuse can occur in any setting, regardless of socioeconomic status. The antecedents of the disorder are not yet clearly defined to provide solutions, and reducing dependency and counterdependency would require substantial amounts of money for a large number of low-income families. It also would be no guarantee of success. Institutionalization is likewise no guarantee of reducing the abuse of the elderly.

Reducing the incidence of alcoholism and other substance abuse might also reduce the risk of elder abuse. These goals are being pursued by a number of agencies, and their achievement would reduce the prevalence of many other social ills as well. Achieving a job market for all working-age people might solve indigency and dependency problems.

A more realistic approach to prevention would be providing a support system for the caregiver and better education. Examples include inservice programs for nursing home personnel, discussion of alternative methods for dealing with behavioral problems, and providing a forum for sharing of ideas, problems, and stories. The importance of support groups and social services are discussed in other chapters. However, the best hope, for prevention of abuse is in reducing the degree of physical and/or mental impairment in the patient. Allowing the elderly to continue independent living in their own homes by treating potentially debilitating illnesses shows promise.

BIBLIOGRAPHY

Block MR and Sinnott JD, editors: The battered elder syndrome: exploratory study, College Park, 1979, Center on Aging, University of Maryland.

Clark CB: Geriatric abuse—out of the closet, J Tenn Med Assoc 77:470-471, 1984.

Council on Scientific Affairs: Elder abuse and neglect. JAMA 257(7):966-971, 1987.

Elder abuse: a national disgrace. Report by the Subcommittee on Health and Long-term Care of the Select Committee on Aging. US House of Representatives Committee Publication. U.S. Congress, pp 99-502, 1985.

Fulmer TT and O'Malley TA, editors: Inadequate care of the elderly—a health care perspective on abuse and neglect, New York, 1987, Springer Publishing Co, Inc.

Hickey T and Douglass RL: Mistreatment of the elderly in a domestic setting: exploratory study, Am J Public Health 71(5):500-507, 1981.

Kempe CH et al: The battered-child-syndrome, JAMA 181:17-24, 1962.

Sanford, JRA: Tolerance of debility in elderly dependants by supporters at home: its significance for hospital practice, Br Med J 3:471-473, 1975.

O'Malley TA et al: Identifying and preventing family mediated abuse and neglect of elderly persons, Ann Intern Med 98:998-1005, 1983.

Pillemer K and Wolf R: Elder abuse: conflict in the family, Dover, Mass, 1986, Auburn House Publishing Co.

AVAILABLE RESOURCES

16

Support groups for relatives

M. Lancaster, E. Patrick, and B. Abernathy

The entire family, not just the patient, is the unit of concern in the management of Alzheimer's disease. This is especially true when the patient can no longer participate in health care decisions. The various Alzheimer's disease family support groups are one of the major mechanisms used in the management of the disease.

Support groups have a long history of providing mutual aid to their members through the sharing of common experiences and problems. Emotional and social bonds develop between people who participate in support groups because of their similar experiences. If members of a support group are given emotional and social support and are allowed to discuss problems openly and to share joys, the physical and mental strain on the caregivers can be eased, and this may allow the family to provide in-home care for a longer period. A study conducted at Duke University in the early 1980s has demonstrated that the mere feeling of being supported had a greater impact on reducing caregiver strain than the amount of actual outside help (support) the caregiver received.

Most support groups spring from families' need to receive information and emotional assistance. Through education, sharing, guidance, and advocacy, these groups help to increase the family members' confidence in themselves as caregivers. Families have the right to expect to be supported in their caregiving activities. Because no one individual possesses all the knowledge or answers to Alzheimer's disease, the support group serves as an open educational forum for both family members and interested health professionals. This format allows everyone to learn from one another. Additionally, support groups provide the time needed for relaxed, informal discussion and problem solving.

The participants of a support group have varying roles within their community and their own families. However, the common caregiving experience places the group members on a similar level. The members of a group receive support and guidance from one another while lending support and guidance to others. In view of the varying and changing roles of caregivers, a structural aspect of support groups to be considered is the caregiver-patient relationship. Any group may have a mixture of spouses, children, and siblings, each having a unique relationship with the patient. These varying relationships give rise to very different needs, viewpoints, and emotions on the part of the caregivers and the patient. Separate groups currently are being formed specifically to help meet the needs of children or spouses of patients with Alzheimer's disease. Having separate groups can help avoid a potentially disturbing situation in which the spouse and adult child of a patient are in attendance at the same meeting. In this instance the freedom to express true feelings and emotions may be hindered by the presence of another family member.

Health care professionals, who may or may not have personal experience with family members who have Alzheimer's disease, become involved in support groups. When professionals participate, they can lend informational and administrative support to the group. The tasks of phone calls, program planning, and mailings are time consuming, and professionals can assist by taking over responsibility for these tasks. Because health care professionals may not be directly involved with the day-to-day care of someone with Alzheimer's disease, they can also serve as a buffer or sounding board for the group members. These professionals can also lend their expertise and knowledge at the meetings.

It is essential that someone assume the facilitator/moderator position for the group. Groups without designated leaders tend to dissolve within a very short time. The leader takes responsibility for ensuring participation and may call members who fail to show up. This leadership position can be assumed by either a health professional or a family member.

The participants of any support group will work through various stages of involvement in the group. Initially, the interactions may be superficial and evolve around telling one's own story. As basic trust and understanding develop between the members, the group begins to grow and mature and the caregivers begin recognizing and discussing their personal feelings and needs. Eventually this type of discussion enables the members to assist each other in identifying and resolving problems, feelings, and conflicts. This is the ultimate goal of a support group.

The format or structure of a group varies, depending on the size of the group and the needs of the group members. Many groups have a formal structure, which tends to work better for larger groups, and use educational presentations as the major emphasis of the meetings. Other groups are small and informal and may not have any particular agenda for the meeting. In general, the smaller the group, the more quickly trust and openness will develop. In our experiences with support groups, it has been found that during the early stages of group development, it is useful to have a program (e.g., speaker, film) to help ease the tension. Gradually the programs can give way to open discussions on a certain topic or simply to finding out how the members are getting along.

Finally, support groups are a socialization time for the caregivers. Isolated by the necessity to be with their family member 24 hours a day, the social needs of many caregivers frequently are not met. The support group offers a time to meet new people, to develop friendships, and to talk with others who are knowledgeable about Alzheimer's disease. Having the focus of the meeting evolve around the care of the patient can help ease the guilt a caregiver may feel of having taken time for herself.

Support groups provide caregivers a time to bring before a panel of "experienced people" a new problem they have encountered. Caregivers also attend the group meetings because they need to share their tales and share what they have discovered. This sharing helps them to feel as if they can help someone else. Following are some of one of the authors' thoughts on the meaning of support groups to caregivers:

One of the things I discovered was why my mother was not drinking her cranberry juice. I had put it in a green, translucent glass, and it looked like prune juice. I poured it into a clear glass, and she resumed drinking it. She did not like prune juice . . .

When we (caregivers) go to a support group, we shed the image that some people have of us as saints or poor things. We become people who have a common problem . . .

When a couple of people do not come to the meeting for a few months, I wonder how they are doing. I feel like hugging them when I see them. It is like a sisterhood or brotherhood. There is a bond between us that is so important . . .

It has been my experience that my mother's physician is learning from me. He has learned from us to help another patient . . .

We learn how to be nurses from each other. We learn about devices that we can use. We can tap the brains of professionals. Support groups are a social time with a focus . . .

They say that misery loves company. But you do not go to a support group because you are miserable. You go because you have some hope, not that there is a cure, but that there is a way out of your current problems . . .

DANGERS OF SUPPORT GROUPS

Although support groups have been shown to increase the caregiver's sense of support and knowledge about Alzheimer's disease and community resources, there are potential dangers in support groups. Of primary concern is that some support groups may begin to view themselves as a replacement or substitution for professional psychotherapy. Support groups are neither the place nor the mechanism for professional counseling or psychotherapy. However, through a caregiver's interactions and participation in a group, individuals who are experiencing a great amount of stress or difficulty in coping can be identified and referred for professional help.

A second potential danger is one of dependency, either on the group itself or on the leader of the group. In the event the group disbands, caregivers who have become totally dependent on the group for information, social interaction, and support may find themselves at a great loss. This sort of dependency also can focus on the leader of the group. Because of their high visibility in the group, their interest in combating Alzheimer's disease, and their knowledge of the disease, leaders are primary targets to take on the "responsibility" of the other group members. Many group leaders have said that a great deal of time and energy are expended on the problems and needs of other caregivers. This can be especially dangerous if the group leader is also a caregiver; one whose time and energy are already stressed to the maximum. This additional responsibility can lead to burnout of the leader, thus leaving the group members stranded. Through careful guidance, group members can be helped to find additional sources of support outside the group.

Sometimes group members become so familiar with the behavior, problems, and symptoms of the disease that they tend to forget the individual nature of Alzheimer's disease and start packaging information and solutions. Yet this type of "packaged" information may not apply in another person's situation. Along with this familiarity comes the potential to begin diagnosing friends and relatives and to start recommending treatment plans without a proper medical evaluation and diagnostic workup.

When a group has met for an extended period, a great deal of freedom, trust, and understanding develops in the group. The members talk openly about problems and what may be ahead of them. This is one goal of the group, but it must be kept in mind that newcomers may be present at the meeting. New members of the group, especially if their family member has only recently been diagnosed, become easily frightened when hearing about the problems of caregivers and patients dealing with late stages of Alzheimer's disease. They may become so overwhelmed with fear and distaste for the group that they never return. One possible solution is the development of a group for newcomers. These new group members can meet with an especially sensitive caregiver while the "older" group members continue with their discussions. It is a fine line to walk in trying to meet all the needs of caregivers who are experiencing various stages of the disease at the same time.

It is important that group leaders have training in group process. Situations arise that may be very disruptive to the group. Some individuals talk so much that they manipulate the entire time, whereas others never get the chance to speak. Arguments may develop, and some members may appear particularly hostile or abusive. Involving group leaders in workshops on group process can help them feel more comfortable with their role and more assured in handling difficult situations. Additionally, professionals who are experienced in group process can be called upon to assist in the meetings.

Developing, implementing, and running support groups can be stressful and time consuming. Yet there is great satisfaction to be found for those who take on this responsibility. Support groups are for the members. Involving caregivers in a useful and helpful interaction with one another yields personal rewards for everyone. Support groups are not the complete answer to the problems of caregivers, but when combined with appropriate health care follow-up and community resource support, they can be one of the most important tools for success available to the caregiver.

BIBLIOGRAPHY

Davis J: Support groups: a clinical intervention for families of the mentally impaired elderly, J Gerontol Soc Work 5(4):27-35, 1983.

Given CW, Collins CE, and Given BA: Sources of stress among families caring for relatives with Alzheimer's disease, Nurs Clin North Am 23(1):69-82, 1988.

Glasser G and Wexler D: Participants' evaluations of educational/support groups for families of patients with Alzheimer's disease and other dementias, Gerontologist 25(3):232-236, 1985.

Gwyther L: Caregiver self-help groups: roles for professionals, Generations 53:37-38, 1982.

Haley W, Brown S, and Levine E: Experimental evaluation of the effectiveness of group intervention for dementia caregivers, Gerontologist 27(3):376-382, 1987.

Hartford M and Parsons R: Uses of groups with relatives of dependent older adults, Social Work With Groups 5(2):77-89, 1982.

Hayter J: Helping families of patients with Alzheimer's disease, J Gerontol Nurs 8(2):81-86, 1982.

Lecso PA: Murder-suicide in Alzheimer's disease, J Am Geriatr Soc 37(2):167-168, 1989.

Ory MG et al: Families, informal supports, and Alzheimer's disease. Current research and future agendas, Res Aging 7(4):623-644, 1985.

Roberts BL and Algase DL: Victims of Alzheimer's disease and the environment, Nurs Clin North Am 23(1):83-93, 1988.

Shibal-Champagne S, Lipinska-Stachow DM: Alzheimer's educational/supportive group: considerations for success—awareness of family tasks, pre-planning, and active professional facilitation, J Gerontol Soc Work 9(2):41-48, 1985/1986.

17

Social services available

P. Brown

Because Alzheimer's disease is a slow, insidious disorder, caregivers often become more and more involved in caring for their patient and forget to look to the social support system provided by their community. As the patient with Alzheimer's disease gradually deteriorates, the demands on the caregivers gradually increase, until the situation becomes unbearable. Also, not infrequently caregivers are embarrassed to seek the help that may be available. They may have had no experience with social services and may equate them with "being on welfare." On the other hand, they may resent strangers entering their homes or feel that by involving a social agency, they are being disloyal to their spouse or parent.

It is imperative for health professionals to know of the social services available to the elderly. Often when people seek help, they are confused about where to go. One resource readily available for such help is the Area Agency on Aging. The federal agency, The Administration on Aging (AOA) distributes money provided through Title III of the Older Americans Act to each state based on the number of residents 60 years of age or older. The state units on aging then distribute the funds to each Area Agency on Aging, with the proviso that the money be used solely for the benefit of people 60 years of age or older, with emphasis on serving those in greatest social and economic need. There is no charge for programs under the Older Americans Act; however, everyone is encouraged to help defray the cost of services so as to make them more available. Although each Area Agency on Aging is autonomous, certain services for the homebound elderly usually are available in most communities. These include home-delivered meals, a homemaker program, chore services, transportation, legal care, and senior center services, which may include telephone reassurance, friendly visiting, and so forth.

A case management program has become the point of entry for Title III services for the frail, health-impaired elderly. An information and referral specialist makes a home visit to determine what services are necessary to enable that person to remain in his or her home. A care plan is developed and approved under the guidance of a case manager, services are ordered, and a follow-up phone call is made to determine whether the service(s) are being received. Reassessments are conducted every 6 months to verify continued need. The case management program can also arrange for other non-Title III services if requested.

NUTRITION PROGRAM

A few years after the Older Americans Act was passed in 1965, a nutrition program for the elderly was started. Eligibility for the program was based solely on age 60 years or older. Since that time the nutrition program has become the largest component of services delivered through the Area Agency on Aging network. Both congregate and home-delivered programs, operating out of senior citizens centers and, in a few cases, community buildings, are funded. There are local programs that provide emergency food. Probably one of the most helpful programs is the home-delivered meal program. This is a federally funded program that is coordinated with church-sponsored, meals-on-wheels programs in local cities. Meals are prepared and packed in a central kitchen and delivered by volunteers. The nutrition program provides meals for the homebound 5 days a week, and although special diets are not available, the menus meet low-sodium requirements and provide one third of the required daily dietary allowance.

A complete assessment is performed to establish need for meals, and the spouse of a participant may receive a meal if it is deemed to be in the couple's best interest. The Administration on Aging also recently approved homebound meals for the adult dependent child of a frail, homebound elderly person who receives the meal. Area agencies have devised various ways to provide meals to as many people as possible. For those who live in remote areas, a packet of five frozen meals may be delivered by a volunteer once a week or every 5 days if the person is also in need of weekend meals. The client is also given a toaster oven if there is no oven in the home.

OTHER SERVICES

Next to home-delivered meals, the homemaker program is one of the most important services for the frail, health-impaired elderly. The homemaker may do house cleaning, laundry, grocery shopping, run errands, meal preparation and, in some cases, personal care. Limited funding makes this service available on the average of twice a month. However, sometimes it is possible to receive weekly homemaker services on a temporary basis to assist in a recuperation. The homemaker program also tries to provide volunteers for shopping and errands, which frees the homemaker's time for cleaning, laundry, and so forth. Chore services may include heavy cleaning and outdoor chores such as bringing in wood and coal and yard work. Minor home repairs are also done through the use of volunteers for labor. Clients are asked to buy the necessary supplies, but if they are not able to do so the program attempts to get donated supplies. Repairs for steps, construction of a wheelchair ramp, and replacement of window and door screens are examples of the minor repairs that can be completed. Probably the most difficult request received is for roof repairs, but if the roof needs to be replaced, the individual will be referred to a reputable company in the hope that the firm will perform the work at a reduced fee.

Related to home repairs is the weatherization program, which usually is funded through another agency. But because the programs so often serve the same people, the agencies try to coordinate the work. This program provides income-eligible people with storm windows and insulation for their homes.

Interest-free loans may be available from local utility companies to anyone, regardless of age or income, who wants to upgrade their homes to make them more energy efficient. Nearly all utility companies have another program that benefits individuals on a fixed income: a budget billing plan, which allows participants to pay an average amount each month with an adjustment once a year.

TRANSPORTATION

In nearly all assessments conducted to determine the needs of older people, transportation is usually at the top of the list. However, the kinds of transportation available are as diverse as the communities themselves. Some districts have rural mass transit programs that are based in the senior center in each county. Two-way radios enable the dispatchers to operate vans in an efficient manner. Reasonable fares are charged to riders, regardless of age. Most of the vans are equipped with wheelchair lifts, and the drivers are trained in transporting handicapped people for doctor's appointments and so forth. It should be noted, however, that the vans do not have oxygen and are not a substitute for ambulances. There are also some agencies and organizations that provide transportation. For example, the Department of Human Services pays for transportation services for some low-income people who are receiving public benefits. The American Cancer Society and the American Kidney Foundation will provide volunteer transportation to treatment centers. Information on these programs may be obtained from the pertinent treatment centers or from the local offices of the Department of Human Services.

HOME HEALTH CARE

A phenomenon of the 1980s is the rapid growth of home health care agencies. Some area agencies contract for home nursing visits for those people who may not have Medicare or Medicaid. All home nursing services, however, require a physician's orders, whether paid for by Medicare, Medicaid, Title III, or private insurance. Currently, Medicaid pays for 60 home visits in 1 year. Effective Jan. 1, 1990, Medicare will cover up to 6 days a week of intermittent home health care and up to 38 continuous days in any given period. In-home care of up to 80 hours per year will be provided for a chronically dependent person who meets the catastrophic limits or the prescription drug deductible.

INSURANCE

One of the most confusing issues an elderly person or caregiver has to contend with is health insurance. The insurance industry is in a state of flux, with the long-term care policy being the most recent innovation. Long-term care coverage is limited and very specific, and people are advised to choose carefully. As a general rule, the younger a person is when purchasing such a policy, the lower the premium. After the age of 60, the premium increases dramatically. Some policies pay the full nursing home rate the first month but reduce the amount thereafter. Currently most policies are limited to 6-year coverage, and many do not have a built-in factor to offset the inflationary increases in costs.

Medicare is a health insurance program sponsored by the federal government for people 65 years of age or older, as well as certain disabled people. Medicaid is a program funded by both the state and federal governments to provide health care for low-income people. Those who are on Medicare may or may not want supplemental insurance, but it is important to remember that an older person who is covered by Medicaid needs no other insurance. (Note: Under the new Medicare Catastrophic Coverage Act, Medicaid will pay the Medicare premium for a Supplemental Security Income [SSI] recipient, thus providing the SSI recipient with increased coverage).

Since insurance is so complicated, it is advisable to call the local Social Security office or the local office of the Department of Human Services to get the latest, most accurate information. The importance of being well-informed when making decisions on insurance needs cannot overemphasized. Although older adults make up only 12% of the U.S. population today, they constitute 60% of the victims of health care fraud.

BENEFITS

Aside from Social Security and SSI benefits, there are other forms of public benefits such as food stamps, tax relief, property tax exemptions, local utility discounts, and sometimes discounts at participating stores. Members of the American Association of Retired Persons (AARP) also receive discounts at participating businesses and can order prescription drugs at a reduced cost. An AARP annual membership is well worth the $5 it costs, especially for those who are on maintenance drugs. Those who meet income guidelines are eligible for food commodities, as well as assistance with energy bills, through the U.S. Department of Health and Human services Low Income Energy Assistance Program (LIEAP). There are also veterans and railroad pensions, as well as private retirement and pension plans. It sometimes takes a little detective work to uncover all benefits due to an older person. The case management staff of the Area Agency on Aging is trained to assist the homebound elderly in obtaining these benefits.

LEGAL SERVICES

Area agencies contract with attorneys to provide legal care for older people, and they also arrange for the services of a long-term care ombudsman. Assistance with legal problems is needed by everyone at some time in his or her life, and the lack of such help can be a source of great irritation and despair. This program provides assistance in all legal matters, including administrative hearings on denial of benefits, property disputes, and the like.

The long-term care ombudsman is one who serves as an advocate for nursing home residents. The ombudsman provides information to families regarding long-term care facilities and can assist in making nursing home arrangements. The ombudsman also receives and investigates complaints from a resident or the resident's family regarding the facility in which the patient is located. The ombudsman serves in an advocacy role while trying to achieve equitable resolutions to problems, report findings in a confidential manner, and identify needed improvements in the facilities. In some states a volunteer ombudsman program is being developed. These volunteers are assigned to one or two facilities and must commit to making visits at least once a month. The volunteer may not resolve a complaint but reports any findings to the ombudsman, who then handles the complaint in the appropriate manner.

SAFETY DEVICES

One of the greatest fears of many elderly people is that they will fall and break a bone and that no one will find them until it is too late. There are several safety devices that enable frail, elderly people to remain in their homes with a certain degree of reassurance that someone will be checking on them. Today, there are several emergency response systems on the market. With most systems the individual buys a unit to be placed in the home, pays a monthly fee, and is linked by phone to a base station, which is usually located in a hospital. The individual may alert the base station by pressing a "panic button."

Some security businesses have response systems in addition to burglar systems. There is a "Red-Eye Alert" program operated by local fire departments that will provide, upon request, a "red-eye" sticker that is placed on the door or front of the house. If there is a fire, the firefighter is alerted to the fact that there is an invalid in the house who will need assistance. A familiar program, the "Vial of Life," is a project of the AARP. This organization will furnish anyone with a plastic container in which to place pertinent medical information. The container is placed in the refrigerator, and a sticker is placed on the front door indicating that there is a vial of life in the home.

Another program is the Carrier Alert Program. Participating individuals have a sticker on their mailbox, and if the postal carrier notices that mail is not being picked up, he notifies his supervisor, who then calls the senior citizens center to send someone to check on the individual. The Gatekeeper Program is yet another program that alerts utility meter readers to notice conditions around the home of an elderly person that might indicate the person is experiencing difficulties. Most senior citizens centers will make daily telephone calls, if requested, to be sure a homebound person is all right. In addition to all these emergency services, most cities now have a 911 telephone emergency number that receives and handles distress calls.

RESPITE/HOSPICE DAY CARE

Respite and hospice day care are programs that are fairly new in the field of social services. Informal respite exists in small communities where people live in close contact with their neighbors. A neighbor is willing to "run over and sit" with a patient while the caregiver goes to the grocery store or on an errand. This is a simple form of respite care. Hospital and nursing homes provide overnight, weekend or longer respite care for caregivers who wish to go out of town but are unable to leave their patient unattended. However, this is usually private pay and very expensive. Volunteer respite programs have sprung up but are only as successful as the dedication of the person is running the program. It is difficult to get a "match" between the patient and the volunteer, as quite often the patient does not accept a stranger. Also, the caregiver, especially one whose patient has Alzheimer's disease, is reluctant to trust the volunteer with the patient.

Hospice care is a fairly new service. Care may be provided either in a hospital or a home setting. Medicare will reimburse for hospice care only in approved programs. (Note: The Medicare Catastrophic Coverage Act provides for unlimited hospice care, in approved programs, as long as the physician states the need exists.)

Adult day care, geriatric day care, or dependent day care are all terms used to describe programs in which the patient with Alzheimer's disease is cared for during the day. In some states there are no licensure requirements, so great care should be exercised in placing a person in a day care program. Relatives should check to be sure that the program meets all local fire, safety, and health codes and that the staff has good credentials. Adult day care enables many caregivers to continue working if their patient is fairly mobile. Many programs, however, will not accept patients who are incontinent.

HOUSING ALTERNATIVES

Sooner or later most caregivers are faced with the situation of no longer being able to cope with the demands of the patient living in the home or with the caregiver. At this juncture a decision must be made about alternative housing arrangements. There are several housing facilities that provide different levels of care. Some facilities accept a person who is well and able to live independently, offering the promise of congregate dining, housekeeping services, and eventually a nursing home bed. Some facilities also monitor medications, thus delaying nursing home placement. Some facilities offer both skilled and unskilled nursing care, whereas others offer only unskilled care. Some nursing homes have special Alzheimer's units, but the cost, which in today's circumstances is private pay, is almost double that of an intermediate-care facility. All facilities should meet state and local licensure requirements.

SENIOR CITIZENS CENTERS

No report on services to the elderly would be complete without mention of senior citizens centers. Although these centers have been referred to throughout the description of services, it needs to be emphasized that they are recognized community focal points for services listed. Others are geared to serving active, independent older people. All are informed about the availability of services for senior citizens and should be looked on as a source when determining how to meet the needs of the elderly.

SUMMARY

The process of getting an elderly person and/or his family to agree to seek help may be even more difficult than locating the needed services. It requires not only a great deal of patience, understanding, and compassion, but also a thorough working knowledge of the services available. For specific information on what services for the elderly are available in a particular area, the local senior citizens center or Area Agency on Aging, both of which are listed in the yellow pages of most telephone directories, should be contacted directly. If there is no senior center or agency on aging in the area, the state office on aging is a resource.

BIBLIOGRAPHY

A profile of older Americans, Washington, D.C., 1986, American Association of Retired Persons.

Commonwealth Fund Commission on Elderly People Living Alone, Baltimore, Ma, 1987.

Marshall JY: Dental care and the older adult, Aging Network News, Bethesda, Md, 1987, Omni Reports, Ltd.

Statewide study of the needs of senior Tennesseans, Nashville, Tenn, 1986, First Tennessee District, Tennessee Commission on Aging.

18

The role of the nurse in an Alzheimer's unit

M. Lancaster and J. Broome

Nurses who work on the Alzheimer's unit of a nursing home or some other institution have many functions, including coordinating communication, teaching, and helping the patient to stay as healthy as possible.

THE NURSE AS COMMUNICATOR AND COORDINATOR

As a communicator and coordinator, the nurse deals with the patient, the patient's relatives, previous caregivers, other nursing staff (including auxillary nursing staff and volunteer workers), rehabilitation therapists, social workers, the physician, the administrative staff of the nursing home, and all others who are involved with the patient. Being an effective communicator and coordinator requires certain qualities such as being a good listener and being able both to gather information from a wide range of sources and to update the information as often as required. A good communicator and coordinator encourages others to share their information and ensures that an adequate mechanism exists for collecting this information. The nurse must have all the data relating to the patient to form a clear, comprehensive picture of the patient's physical, mental, and social condition. Without this information constantly at her fingertips, the nurse can quickly lose credibility as a communicator and source of current patient information.

Finally, an effective communicator ensures that information is conveyed effectively whether or not she is present. To achieve this, a mechanism for collecting and disseminating information must be established. It is important, therefore, to formulate a comprehensive patient assessment to provide a picture of the patient's progress and/or problems and the care to be provided. An incomplete nursing assessment can only generate confusion and an inappropriate plan of care.

All members of the health care team should contribute to the assessment. Nursing assistants have an important role as team members, because they may be more aware of some of the patient's problems that may have escaped the attention of other team members. It is also paramount to involve the patient's relatives.

A great deal can be learned from families who have cared for their loved one long before the person required nursing home care. Information must be collected from the family, since the patient often is unable to relate a good history. Data collected from the family should include information about the patient's vocabulary, what certain words mean, and what certain behavioral patterns indicate. These patterns should be known and documented, so that all staff members are aware of them.

It is important to find out about the patient's life-style before admission to the nursing home. Inquiries should be made about hobbies, special interests, food preferences, and what is considered normal for the patient's bowel and bladder functions. Inquiries should also be made about problems that arose at home before the patient was admitted to the nursing home and the family's means of managing them. If a particular approach to a specific problem was effective in the home situation, this approach is also likely to be appropriate in the nursing home. The relationship between the patient's family and the nursing home staff may be influenced by interpersonal problems that existed before the patient was placed in the nursing home or that arose subsequently. Such problems as the financial burden of caring for a relative and disposing of family property may influence the family's behavior while visiting in the nursing home. Many family members feel a sense of guilt or even shame at having placed their relative in an institution.

If staff members are aware of problems within the family, they can better understand the behavior of the patient and family, can be more tolerant of their behavior, and can be of help to the family.

The importance of good nursing notes cannot be overemphasized; they are the most effective method of conveying vital information to all caregivers. Updating the plan of care is essential for continuity of care, and regular case conferences are another essential. Such conferences are necessary to formulate an appropriate management plan and to reevaluate both patient care needs and the plan of care. Weekly meetings promote improved patient care, a more informed family, and optimum use of resources.

A thorough nursing assessment, including a medical history, should be performed on admission to the nursing home. It is important to find out about any other diagnoses the patient may have, as other medical conditions may be responsible for mental, clinical, or nursing problems at a later stage. Furthermore, whenever communicating with the primary care physician, it is important to remind him or her of the patient's medical diagnoses, as these may alter the physician's management plan. The physician may not have access to the patient's records all the time, so relating the patient's name, the presenting problem, and other known diagnoses helps the physician formulate an appropriate plan of care more quickly and accurately.

The nurse must also clinically examine the patient; this data may be collected according to anatomical systems. Vital signs, disabilities, contractures, and breaks in the skin should be included in this assessment. The results of the assessment, including both positive and negative findings, should be documented on admission. This assessment should be updated on a regular basis and should include changes in vital signs, weight, and nursing care plans. Any pertinent psychological or sociological history must also be included in the documentation.

As the medical condition of nursing home patients with Alzheimer's disease is usually stable, there is no need for a physician to be physically present in the facility all the time. However, there are times when it is very important for the nurse to perform assessments on the patient and to call the physician, communicating as much relevant information about the patient as possible. The more knowledgeable the nurse is about the patient's condition, the more pertinent is the information that is communicated. This in turn promotes earlier intervention, adequate, timely treatment, and an appropriate plan of care.

THE NURSE AS TEACHER

The professional nurse in the role of a teacher is responsible for the continuing education of other nurses and also of the nonprofessional members of the health care team. Continuing education helps to prevent burnout. Obtaining current, short articles about Alzheimer's disease or other diseases that the patient may have and sharing these during informal conferences help keep the minds of the various team members alert, promote interest in patient care, and encourage the team to look for ways to improve the care provided.

Short in-service education sessions should be planned regularly, and as many people as possible should be allowed to attend. If staff members are working on other tours of duty, attempts should be made to arrange the hours for in-service to include them. A discussion of the role of the nurse in educating family members can be found in Chapter 13.

THE NURSE AS MAXIMIZER OF THE PATIENT'S HEALTH

Application of nursing procedures includes administering medication, applying dressings, bowel and bladder training programs, physical exercise, and other measures that promote a state of wellness. Many of these responsibilities may overlap with the duties of other team members, especially the physical and occupational therapists. It is imperative that the nursing staff and the therapists work together in these areas. It is also important to do as much with the patient as time allows.

The likelihood of a patient developing a urinary tract infection can be reduced by increasing the oral fluid intake and by promoting adequate emptying of the bladder. If the patient is ambulatory, he should be encouraged to go to the bathroom as often as possible, since this promotes complete emptying of the bladder. In a prone position, it is difficult to adequately empty the bladder, thereby producing urinary stasis, which predisposes to urinary tract infections. Indwelling Foley catheters also predispose to urinary tract infections (this is further discussed in Chapter 11). For most patients, therefore, the external catheter might be the best approach when a drainage device is needed.

Preventing decubitus ulcers is very important. Adequate diet, good skin care, keeping the skin dry, and frequent changes in position are the basics of decubitus prevention. The patient should be up and around as much as possible. However, when a patient is confined to a bed, turning him every 2 hours helps relieve undue pressure. If the patient is confined to a wheelchair, he can use his arms to push himself up and momentarily relieve pressure on the buttocks.

Use of pneumovaccine and influenza vaccine in nursing home patients contributes to reducing the incidence of pneumonia. Currently it is recommended that the pneumovaccine be administered only once, as this is considered adequate for a lifetime. The influenza vaccine, on the other hand, provides a shorter-lived protection and should be given annually. Since upper respiratory tract infections and pneumonia often complicate influenza, it is felt that use of the influenza vaccine reduces the incidence of these infections. The nurse must collaborate with the physician in ordering and administering these vaccines at the appropriate times.

Preventing falls is extremely important because of the high incidence of complications associated with falls, such as hip fractures. Patients are at risk of falls because of unsteady gait and the inability to understand that there is danger in certain areas. Sometimes the patient's sense of direction is not clear, and this may contribute to repeated falls. Providing supervised and assisted ambulation, if possible, can help reduce the incidence of falls while maintaining mobility.

SUMMARY

Nurses who function in the various roles just described help patients to maximize their capabilities and minimize their limitations. In patients suffering from Alzheimer's disease, every attempt should be made to prevent physical deterioration and to maintain the current level of functioning. The focus of care of the patient with Alzheimer's disease is on maintenance and prevention through a coordinated team effort. Patients and family members often view nurses as people who soothe, console, and relieve stress. However, the nurse's role is much more far reaching and is a vital part of the management of the patient.

BIBLIOGRAPHY

Beck C and Heacock P: Nursing interventions for patients with Alzheimer's disease, Nurs Clin North Am 23(1):95-124, 1988.

Buckwalter KC, Abraham IL, and Neundorfer MM: Alzheimer's disease. Involving nursing in the development and implementation of health care for patients and families, Nurs Clin North Am 23(1):1-9, 1988.

19

Roles of the physical therapist, occupational therapist, and recreation therapist

M. Grossman

The use of physical, occupational, and recreational therapists in the care and treatment of patients with Alzheimer's disease frequently are limited by the accessibility of such therapists, financial coverage for services, and a lack of understanding as to what the therapist can add to the patient/family treatment plan. The services of therapists are not always available locally, and Medicare does not cover these services for a patient with a primary diagnosis of Alzheimer's disease. This is unfortunate, because consultation with therapists can be of great benefit to caregivers at various stages of the disease.

The basis for Medicare's denial of coverage is that the patient cannot be rehabilitated in traditional terms. In other words, the patient does not make progress and get better. However, learning to adapt to the environment, knowing which safety precautions to take, and learning how to stimulate a person so that he can function in all spheres at as high a level as possible for as long as possible is of great value.

The physical therapist can evaluate the patient's functional ability, especially for mobility and safety while standing, walking, and making transfers. The therapist can recommend consideration of a wheelchair for safe mobility. In general, after an evaluation, a maintenance program can be developed for the patient that prescribes the level of exercise needed to maintain strength and flexibility. The physical therapist can teach proper and safe transfer techniques, not only for the patient but for the caregiver as well.

The physical therapist can also evaluate the patient's gait pattern. Constant movement and pacing are common, as the patient may be searching endlessly for something or someone. Yet problems of gait and balance pose great potential for injury. In the later stages, gait is affected. Two common patterns are a stiff-stooped posture with slow shuffling steps and limited arm movement, or a rapid scissor gait with a forward thrust of the upper body, arms across the chest, moving and grasping at anything or anyone.

The physical therapist can advise the caregiver as to a good exercise program, keeping in mind that active range of motion is much more beneficial than passive. Active range of motion is what the patient does himself, whereas passive range of motion is done to the patient. Active movements can be stimulated by participation in games or other activities. Keeping the patient active, up walking during the day, and exercising as long as possible is most important. It is true that "if they do not use it, they will lose it." An adequate program of exercise and activity during the day also ensures that the patient has a good night's sleep. Once an activity or skill is lost, it will generally not be regained. Although a description of range of motion exercises for the bedridden patient is beyond the scope of this book, each joint should be put through a full range of motion to prevent contractures. Care must be exercised not to cause pain.

Recreational therapists can be found directing activity programs in psychiatric or long-term care facilities and on hospital units. They utilize many means to devise a therapeutic use of recreational activities. The caregiver can learn a great deal from recreational therapists, and if they are not available for direct consultation, many of their "tools" can be used.

Taking a patient with Alzheimer's disease to a new place or on an outing can be very confusing, frustrating, and frightening for both the caregiver and the patient. Although some patients may still want to explore new places, most may feel comfortable going to places that are familiar to them, such as their church or local stores. Trips to stores should be arranged at times when the stores are not crowded. Outings can give relief to the caregiver, but these trips must be well planned. It is extremely important to know the patient, what stage of the disease he is in, and how he reacts to new situations. It is probably wise to have another individual who knows the patient (in addition to the caregiver) go along on any outing. The second person can drive or distract the patient while the caregiver drives.

Crafts that are geared to the patient's level, simple and repetitive but of adult interest, are helpful. The main point to remember is that patients with Alzheimer's disease are adults with a disease that affects their brain and, therefore, their function. They are not children. They have led productive, independent lives and deserve respect. Crafts that utilize old and favored skills can be useful to stimulate brain activity.

Games are also incorporated into therapeutic recreation programs. Patients may remember simple familiar games while forgetting many other things. Games stimulate the mind and provide good use of leisure time. Some games that might be helpful include checkers, dominoes, card games (using large-faced cards), ring toss, bean bag throw, tossing and catching a balloon, picture bingo, tic tac toe, horseshoes, catch with a large softball, or just bouncing a ball.

Dancing and music, especially songs popular in the patient's youth, are valuable and can foster reminiscence therapy. Simple activities such as making cookies also can be fun. Rolling the dough into small balls is easy, and there is no need to worry if the patient puts the dough in his mouth.

Repetitive activities such as raking leaves or vacuuming are easy and simple and make good use of preservation (the tendency to repeat a motion that many patients with Alzheimer's disease exhibit). The main thing that must be remembered is to keep the activity simple. Complex activities that require sorting and using several different skills can produce sensory overload and cause confusion and frustration. Patients can become afraid of a complex activity or one that requires the use of lost skills.

Sports activities are another good outlet. Pool can be played without concern for all the proper rules by just "hitting the ball into the hole at the end of the table." Watching live sports events with someone who will narrate can be a good activity. If attendance at a ball game is planned, the caregiver should be prepared to walk around or to leave early if necessary.

Parties are another good tool of the therapeutic recreator. Parties can trigger a chance to reminisce about birthdays or celebrations of holidays and special festivities. The caregiver can make a scrapbook of pictures of family members and special events in the patient's life. Knowing what the patient liked in the past can guide the caregiver as to what the patient will want to do. A former businessman may enjoy attending meetings, whereas a former trucker might like to take a short trip. Trips to the zoo or amusement park can be useful.

An occupational therapist evaluates the patient to help determine at what level the patient is functioning. In the early stages of Alzheimer's disease, the patient should be checked to see if he can function independently or to assess what degree of supervision is needed for safety. The occupational therapist looks at the whole person and tries to see what is most important to the patient and family.

The occupational therapist also helps the patient achieve the highest level of independent functioning. In patients with Alzheimer's disease, the goal is to *maintain* the level of function for as long as possible. Home skills can be evaluated by an occupational therapist, who can check for safe cooking practices and can suggest written signs to remind the patient to turn off the stove. Work simplification techniques can help patients plan for a simpler life and prepare them, if possible, for what lies ahead. Money management skills and care of the home are also of vital importance.

As the disease progresses, the occupational therapist can evaluate the degree of independence in performing activities of daily living such as self-feeding. Self-feeding involves several steps. Food must be placed in the mouth, chewed, and swallowed. Some patients have problems with filling the mouth too full, or "squirreling" the food (filling the cheeks up and not getting the food down). The patient must recall the steps involved in eating. It should be remembered that liquids are more difficult to swallow than solid foods. The patient should be allowed to do as much as possible for himself and then, when needed, the caregiver can assist or feed him. The more a person can do for himself, the better he will feel about himself.

Finger foods can be used if patients cannot manage utensils. As the disease progresses, patients most likely will require pureed foods. Adaptive equipment that can help the patient remain independent in self-feeding is available, including nonspill cups, scoop dishes with nonskid bottoms, nonskid surfaces, and plate guards.

Another way to help patients maintain self-esteem is to offer them choices; asking if they want a bite of meat or potatoes, or do they want milk or coffee. This can give them a sense of control, but caution must be used not to confuse them. Choices are best offered when there are only two items to choose between. One-step commands and simple yes-no questions are best. It must be remembered that on one day questions and choices might work, and the next day they may not. Most of all, neither patients nor caregivers should become frustrated. Patients may be distracted from the task of eating by being presented with too many choices. Too many plates or too many people at the table. For example, a patient's husband complained that when he took his wife to a restaurant, she never finished her meal. When questioned, he admitted that she always sat facing all the other patrons in the restaurant. When he followed the recommendation that his wife sit with her back to the other customers and face the wall, she had no problems.

Occupational therapists also evaluate functions with regard to personal hygiene such as bathing, cleansing after using the toilet and brushing teeth. Sometimes patients just need written reminders posted in prominent places; other times verbal cues are required. Frequently just telling the patient what to do next helps. Other times, they will need physical assistance by getting them started in the motion or by demonstrating it first. Although it may be easier simply to do something for the patient, it is better for him to do as much as possible for himself.

Dressing skills include being able to put on clothes and take them off and managing buttons, snaps, zippers, and belts. Also important in dressing is being able to select clothing appropriately, not only as to what matches, but also what is appropriate for the weather and the occasion. The occupational therapist might recommend some clothing adaptations using Velcro and elastic shoelaces.

Other skills that the occupational therapist works on are grooming, money management, and writing. Grooming skills include makeup, hair care, and self-shaving. For example, the patient may have used a straight-edged razor all his life, so it may be hard to persuade him to change. However, switching to an electric razor allows him to manage his own shaving safely. Money management skills include being able to make change, balancing the checkbook, paying bills on time, and making only sensible purchases. Writing skills must also be assessed. The patient may become very repetitive in writing. When a person can no longer sign a check, he has lost much of the control over his financial life.

The occupational therapist can also suggest means of sensory stimulation for the patient. This becomes especially important for institutionalized patients or those living in one room. For the sense of sight, stimulating and bright colors are most important. Plants and live animals can also be used. For instance, bird feeders could be placed outside the windows. A flower garden is not only good for the sense of sight, the patient might also help tend it. Using textures and shapes are important for stimulating the sense of touch.

The use of pets (pet therapy) in the nursing home or at home is a wonderful way to stimulate all the senses. There are many reports of people who were once totally withdrawn becoming socially active after the introduction of pets. If the patient had a favorite pet at home, efforts should be made to arrange for visits with the pet. Family members can be encouraged to bring the pet for a visit. However, a few precautions should be kept in mind when instituting pet therapy. The patients should be screened to assure that there are no fears of house pets, and the interactions of pets and patients need to be observed to make sure that the demented patient does not become abusive of the animal. Cats and dogs are the most popular animals used in pet therapy because of their love for people and because they can be held and stroked. Fish and birds can also be used, but they do not provide the hands-on contact that is so valuable.

Physical, occupational, and recreational therapists can lend emotional support and physical assistance to make caring for an impaired person much easier. Their knowledge, expertise, and plans for management help the patient with Alzheimer's disease to function for a longer and more vital period.

BIBLIOGRAPHY

Beam I: Helping families survive, Am J Nurs 84(2):229-232, 1984.

Dorey M: Alzheimer's disease—the "new" old approach, Physical Therapy Forum 4(32):3-5, 1985.

Kiernat JM: Environment: the hidden modality, Phys Occup Ther Geriatr 2:3-12, 1982.

Olin DW: Assessing and assisting the persons with dementia: an occupational behavior perspective, Phys Occup Ther Geriatr 3:25-32, 1985.

Rogers JC: Occupational therapy services for Alzheimer's disease and related disorders (position paper/American Occupational Therapy Association), Am J Occup Ther 40(12):822-824, 1986.

20

Role of orientation therapy and reminiscence therapy

B. Smith

This chapter focuses primarily on the role reality orientation and reminiscence therapy play in stimulating human interaction while reducing confusion and disorientation. Another purpose behind these psychotherapeutic approaches is to minimize the feelings of hopelessness and despair that are commonly associated with social isolation. These approaches may also slow the deterioration of functions so typical of Alzheimer's disease.

Some general principles apply to both reality orientation and reminiscence therapy.

GENERAL PRINCIPLES
Visual Aids

Visual aids compensate for impaired eyesight and include such things as eyeglasses, clocks with large and bold-faced characters, calendars, pictures, and picture labels. Keeping familiar objects or furniture in their accustomed location also provides visual patterns that cue the patient with familiar behavioral responses.

Name Recognition

Name recognition cues the person and promotes self-esteem. Patients should always be addressed by name. When communicating with the patient, caregivers should place themselves on eyelevel or slightly below eyelevel with the patient. When a caregiver stands or is situated in a position over the patient, this gives a subtle message of power and control that can be threatening to the patient with Alzheimer's disease. Caregivers, whether family or professional, should always introduce themselves and explain the purpose of their visit. Professional caregivers should also wear name tags with large, bold-faced printed names.

Time Cues

Besides addressing the person by name, the caregiver should refer to the time of day in her greeting. These simple strategies serve to orient the person to the caregiver's identity and to the time of day without calling attention to the fact.

Verbal Communication

Patients with Alzheimer's disease may react to changes in their daily routine with a variety of behaviors. Anger, refusal to cooperate, anxiety, and tearfulness may all result from a request for the patient to engage in some activity. It is vital that the caretaker remain calm and accepting of the patient's reaction.

Even though the patient may not respond verbally or may appear to be unaware of efforts to communicate, situations and events should be explained in short, clear statements. Speaking clearly is not synonymous with speaking loudly, nor does it imply speaking to an adult as though the patient were 3 years old. The patient with Alzheimer's disease is quite sensitive to touch and the empathic communication of feelings.

Fatigue, overstimulation, inability to meet the expectations of others, and misinterpretation of both behavior and conversation tend to increase overreactive responses by these patients. Recognizing the warning signals of impending overractive outbursts is vital to preventing such outbursts. No therapeutic intervention program such as reality orientation or reminiscence therapy will be effective if the patient is fatigued or overstimulated.

REALITY ORIENTATION

Taulbee and Folsom in 1966 developed the first reality orientation program for profoundly disoriented patients in a Veterans Hospital in Alabama. The major thrust of their intervention strategy was a 24-hour consistent approach using all personnel in contact with the patients. In the 24-hour reality orientation approach, communications and instructions are given in brief sentence structure. Clear, simple words are used. Staff members are taught how and what to communicate in a calm, consistent manner. Personnel are instructed to guide patients to and from their destinations as needed. As a result, routines become dependable and provide the patients with a structured pattern of expectations. In this manner the patient is continuously given information about who he is, where he is, the current date and time of day, and planned activities. An example of the approach follows:

"Mr. Smith, it is now Monday, March 14. This morning the nursing assistant is going to take you to the hospital dining room for breakfast."

Information about the patients' environment as it relates to activities of daily living must also be consistently provided. In this approach the patient is given information about who he is, where he is, the direction he is moving, and the behavioral expectations of the patient associated with that directional movement. Although time orientation is important, every interaction the staff members have with the patient does not need to include the date and time. An example of this type of reality orientation interactions follows:

"John, this is the dining room. See the sign by the door? (pause) This is where you eat all your meals."

Calling attention to the sign on the door helps the patient with environmental orientation. Referring to the purpose of the room in terms of activities of daily living helps the patient create or reestablish a familiar pattern of behavior.

In addition to a 24-hour reality orientation approach, small group interactions in a classroom environment may be used. Reality orientation as originally outlined by Taulbee and Folsom is a total patient care approach grounded in the patient's daily living context. When the approach is used in a supportive group in a classroom environment for 15 to 20 minutes a day, it takes on the added properties of supportive therapy.

When used, classroom reality orientation should be conducted daily at the same time and location. For patients with Alzheimer's disease, the classes should be limited to a maximum of four or five members. In the classes, basic information such as the members' names and the current date and location of the class are presented. A reality orientation board or a chalkboard with the written date and location on it serve as an excellent visual reinforcement tool. The general process to be used in the classroom is as follows:

1. The staff members introduce themselves by name.
2. The procedures that will be followed are presented.
3. Each patient is addressed individually by name, and the topic for discussion is introduced.
4. The staff members wait a few minutes to let the patient have an opportunity to respond. This may take 2 to 3 minutes per person.
5. The process of introducing the topic and waiting for the patient to recall it is repeated until every member of the group is successful (the staff member reads the data when patients are unable to do so).
6. Immediate feedback should be provided to each patient to reinforce accuracy.

As the class progresses, clocks and calendars can also be used to reinforce telling time and naming dates. Sometimes additional data may be used to stimulate cognitive function. For example, "Today is Wednesday, November 23, 1988. It is the day before Thanksgiving." In this manner significant holidays that relate to group member's experiences can also be introduced and used to reinforce present reality.

Many research studies have shown that the results of reality orientation therapy may not be apparent immediately. In addition, there is some evidence that reality orientation helps retard the degenerative processes associated with Alzheimer's disease. Therefore, it is important that the caregivers continue to use the reality orientation approaches consistently, even if results are not readily apparent.

REMINISCENCE THERAPY

Reminiscence is a process of reviewing past events and situations that uses the cognitive function of memory. Reminiscence generally evokes sensations of nostalgia. It has also been described as part of the meaningful life review process that people commonly experience as they grow older.

Reminiscence therapy is an adaptive strategy that compensates for present losses and inadequacies. It serves to promote interpersonal social relationships and attachments between older people and others, and it can also promote positive self-esteem.

Elderly individuals who are cognitively impaired either by Alzheimer's disease or by some other degenerative conditions often retain some remote memories. As a result, activities that stimulate memories of past experiences may serve the beneficial purpose of supporting crumbling self-esteem and may prevent or delay the development of feelings of despair. It is important to note that reminiscence cannot be generated when the senses are overloaded nor when a lost skill is required.

Whenever old memories are brought up and discussed, they are not usually challenged or judged for accuracy. It is helpful to consider memories shared with caregivers as a form of personalized gift. Viewed from this perspective, reminiscences do not threaten the self-esteem or competency of the cognitively impaired individual. Confronting the patient for accurate detail and interpreting the patient's intent in sharing a memory are therefore inappropriate. If family caregivers want to participate in a reminiscing experience with the patient with Alzheimer's disease, it is vital that they be instructed to listen to what is being shared and to accept only what is offered; they must also be reminded not to correct the patient or to request specific details of a past experience. Because one-to-one communication can become extremely intense, group reminiscing tends to be a more positive therapeutic approach to these patients. In addition, group reminiscing tends to stimulate latent memories more than individual interaction.

Reminiscence groups used with patients with Alzheimer's disease should be held consistently in one place and at a consistent time. The group should have a maximum of five patients working with two coleaders. The groups can meet for approximately 30 minutes at a time two to three times in one day. Since reminiscence therapy is an adjunctive form of therapy, the groups can also be conducted on a daily basis. Group members may vary in gender, but as much as possible should be of the same age group.

The goals of reminiscence therapy will vary, depending on the group's nature and structure. The goals of reminiscence therapy with patient's with Alzheimer's disease are primarily to stimulate memories, enhance identity confirmation, elevate self-esteem, and increase behavioral socialization skills.

The role of the coleaders in the reminiscence therapy group is to provide a comfortable, supportive environment conducive to group sharing. In the process of creating this kind of environment, the coleaders must be able to select appropriate props to stimulate latent memories, prompt group members to participate, listen, and recognize all contributory efforts regardless of how small. Whenever feelings of anxiety, anger, grief, guilt, or regret are expressed, the coleaders must be able to accept these as part of the full range of emotions commonly experienced by human beings. As patients discuss painful events, the group leaders need to listen carefully and avoid verbal reassurance.

Instead, the leaders can use touch, if appropriate, and allow time for long pauses without interruption. Acceptance of the expression of these feelings and their validation in the group promotes self-affirmation in group members.

Music, fragrances, food, and objects tend to stimulate reminiscences more effectively than printed charts, photographs, or magazine pictures. Whenever magazine pictures are used, large, brightly colored pictures are more effective than black and white ones. This is probably because of the impaired visual acuity.

An element of trust must exist between the group members and the coleaders before reminiscences will actually occur in a new group. Therefore, the novice leader should not give up if patients do not immediately respond. It may take several sessions over several days before the group members feel comfortable relating an experience in the group context. It is crucial for the group leaders to have patience and to allow sufficient time for the group members to speak before closing a given session. Sometimes the coleaders may briefly share a personal reminiscence to bring latent group memories to the surface for discussion.

Every reminiscence group leader must keep the goals of this type of approach in mind: stimulating memory, enhancing identity confirmation, increasing self-esteem, and improving behavioral socialization skills. In so doing, the leaders should never disapprove of something being brought up or described. Instead, the leader should listen and try to determine the meaning of the situation or event. All memories shift over time and in response to a person's emotions. Because of this the accuracy of a shared memory should never be challenged. The coleaders must maintain the attitudinal approach that no one else will be precisely like any of the group members and that no one else will have exactly paralleled their experiences. Each is unique and worthy of positive recognition.

Reminiscence group leaders can stimulate participation by asking general questions such as, "What do you remember about your first . . .?" or "Remember what it feels like to have cold ice cream sliding down your throat on a hot summer's day?" The group leaders should focus on the reminiscer as the central person in any event being described. "What did you feel about that?" or "How do you feel about that now?" Sometimes patients will perseverate and be unable to move past a particular event. As a consequence, others in the group, including the group leaders may become bored. In those instances the patient can be gently stimulated to move on in the following ways:

"You have told us about the time your father gave you a surprise puppy. Now, tell us what you and your puppy did together." or "This seems to have been a very trying time in your life. What did you do to overcome this?"

When experiences are shared in a group situation, much of the group discussion that follows probably will be spent in clarifying the reminiscer's experiences for the others in the group. It is important, therefore, to allot sufficient time for full descriptions. This is also one of the reasons this technique can be used periodically throughout the day on an inpatient unit.

In summary, reality orientation and reminiscence therapy can effectively preserve the ability of the patient with Alzheimer's disease to perceive and contribute in his environment. Strategies for reality orientation and reminiscence can be used in group or individual settings. The strategies can be used by family and professional caregivers on an individual basis, in adult day treatment centers, and in institutions.

BIBLIOGRAPHY

Adams J: Reminiscence—poor law pride, Geriatr Nur (London) 5(6):22-23, 1985.

Adams J and Rouse T: Reminiscence therapy: the remembrance of times past, Geriatr Nur (London) 5(4):32-34, 1985.

Baines S, Saxby P, and Ehlert K: Reality orientation and reminiscence therapy. A controlled cross-over study of elderly confused people, Br J Psychiatry 151:222-231, 1987.

Berghorn FJ and Schafer DE: Reminiscence intervention in nursing homes: what and who changes? Int J Aging Hum Dev 24(2):113-127, 1986-1987.

Brennan PL and Steinberg LD: Is reminiscence adaptive? Relations among social activity level, reminiscence, and morale, Int J Aging Hum Dev 18(2):99-110, 1983-1984.

Clements DB: Reminiscence: a tool for aiding families under stress, MCN 11(2):114-117, 1986.

Cuesta U: Reminiscence and strategies of performance in rotary pursuit tracking, Percept Mot Skills 68(1):219-226, 1989.

Fuller L: Reminiscence: using memories to improve the quality of care for elderly patients, J Pract Nurs 38(3):30-35, 1988.

Goldwasser AN, Auerbach SM, and Harkins SW: Cognitive, affective, and behavioral effects of reminiscence group therapy on demented elderly, Int J Aging Hum Dev 25(3):209-222, 1987.

Hamner ML: Insight, reminiscence, denial, projection: coping mechanisms of the aged, J Gerontol Nurs 10(2):66-68, 81, 1984.

Hyland DT, Ackerman AM, and Jones RG: Reminiscence and autobiographical memory in the study of the personal past, J Gerontol 43(2):35-39, 1988.

Inverarity J: Sporting reminiscence, Australas Nurses J 11(8):31, 1984.

MacRae I: Growth and development — for elders: reminiscence, an underused nursing resource, Nurs Pap 14(1):48-56, 1982.

Molinari V and Reichlin RE: Life review reminiscence in the elderly: a review of the literature, Int J Aging Hum Dev 20(2):81-92, 1984-1985.

Norris AD and Abu El Eileh MT: Reminiscence groups, Nurs Times 78(32):1368-1369, 1982.

Nyatanga B: Reminiscence therapy in old age, Nurs Stand 25:3(26):34-35, 1989.

Oleson M: Legacies, reminiscence, and ego-integrity, Nurse Educ 14(2):26, 1989.

Parsons CL: Group reminiscence therapy and levels of depression in the elderly, Nurse Pract 11(3):68, 1986.

Perschbacher R: An application of reminiscence in an activity setting, Gerontologist 24(4):343-345, 1984.

Poulton JL and Strassberg DS: The therapeutic use of reminiscence, Int J Group Psychother 36(3):381-398, 1986.

Priefer BA and Gambert SR: Reminiscence and life review in the elderly, Psychiatr Med 2(1):91-100, 1984.

Scates SK, et al: Effects of cognitive-behavioral, reminiscence, and activity treatments on life satisfaction and anxiety in the elderly, Int J Aging Hum Dev 22(2):141-146, 1985-1986.

Sherman E: Reminiscence groups for community elderly, Gerontologist 27(5):569-572, 1987.

Taft LB: Remembering and sharing through poetry writing, Nurse Educ 14(1):37-38, 1989.

Tarman VI: Autobiography: the negotiation of a lifetime, Int J Aging Hum Dev 27(3):171-191, 1988.

Taulbee LR and Folsom JC: Reality orientation for geriatric patients, Hosp Comm Psych 17(5):133-135, 1966.

Thornton S, and Brotchie J: Reminiscence: a critical review of the empirical literature, Br J Clin Psychol 26(Pt 2):93-111, 1987.

Tourangeau A: Group reminiscence therapy as a nursing intervention: an experimental study. Part One AARN News Lett 44(8):17-18, 1988.

Tourangeau A: Group reminiscence therapy as a nursing intervention: an experimental study. Part two AARN News Lett 44(9):29-30, 1988.

Viney LL, Benjamin YN, and Preston C: Mourning and reminiscence: parallel psychotherapeutic processes for elderly people, Int J Aging Hum Dev 28(4):239-249, 1989.

Winters JJ Jr, and Semchuk MT: Retrieval from long-term store as a function of mental age and intelligence, Am J Ment Defic 90(4):440-448, 1986.

Wisner BL, Lombardo JP, and Catalano JF: Rotary pursuit performance as a function of sex, sex-role, and intertrial interval, Percept Mot Skills 66(2):443-452, 1988.

Wright BM and Payne RB: Effects of aging on sex differences in psychomotor reminiscence and tracking proficiency, J Gerontol 40(2):179-184, 1985.

21
Legal issues

M. Mettetal

Almost every family of a patient with Alzheimer's disease must at some point address legal issues. A basic understanding of the provisions of guardianship and conservatorship laws, therefore, is helpful to the family. Familiarity with the durable power of attorney law is also beneficial, since its use is appropriate for patients in the very early stages of Alzheimer's disease. Although specific laws vary from state to state, much of the information presented has general applications. Any person considering guardianship, conservatorship, or power of attorney should consult the laws of the state the patient lives in.

A few states have enacted public guardianship laws. The training that public guardians receive in legal issues and the experience they have gained in obtaining government benefits for their clients enables them to present an overall view of matters of concern to patient's with Alzheimer's disease and their families.

Financial problems often develop with these patients in the early stages of the disease. The patient's checking account may be in a terrible mess; checks are often incorrectly written or not recorded, and addition and subtraction errors are common. Unwise financial decisions also often surface. A patient may give away jewelry, money, or other assets that will be needed for future care. For example, one woman sold her $50,000 home to a recently bankrupted neighbor for a $20,000 unsecured personal note and $5,000 in cash.

In the early stages of Alzheimer's disease, family members are advised to gather all the financial information they can, while the patient is still able to help them. They should ascertain details about real estate holdings; income amounts and sources should be noted; and bank accounts and insurance policies should be located. It would be a wise move to take this information to an attorney and to discuss steps that should be taken immediately and plans that should be made to protect the patient's assets.

Many people are reluctant to go to an attorney's office because of the expected high costs. However, most attorneys have an established hourly fee that they charge for office consultations. This fee is a small price to pay to protect a patient's assets. Anyone with a relative who is suspected of having Alzheimer's disease should seek the advise of an attorney.

REGULAR VERSUS DURABLE POWER OF ATTORNEY

In an article about the legal problems of patients with Alzheimer's disease and their families, the director of Legal Care Projects for the Tennessee Commission on Aging stated that "in all cases in which the patient is capable of executing a contract, efforts should be made to obtain a durable power of attorney." This instrument can eliminate the need to have a guardianship petition filed with the court. The durable power of attorney is such an important document that it should always be discussed with and drawn up by an attorney.

The regular power of attorney, familiar to most people, becomes invalid when the person who granted that power of attorney (the patient) becomes incapable or incompetent. In other words, it ceases to be effective when the need is greatest. On the other hand, the durable power of attorney is specifically designed to continue regardless of the mental or physical disability of the person who executed it. The person appointed in either form is called an attorney-in-fact, though this person does not have to be an attorney. The attorney-in-fact should be a trusted friend or relative. The specific powers granted to the attorney-in-fact should be clearly set out. Decisions concerning the health care of the disabled person can and should be included in the specified powers.

The durable power of attorney gives a tremendous amount of power to one person. In addition, once the subject person is disabled, it cannot be easily revoked. The activities of the attorney-in-fact are not supervised by the court the way guardianships and conservatorships are. Like any other relationship based on trust, room for abuse exists. For this reason very careful study and advice is recommended before using the durable power of attorney. The attorney-in-fact must be carefully chosen.

No matter what the course of the disease, at some point the patient with Alzheimer's disease will no longer be able to sign legal documents or make appropriate decisions. Yet bills have to be paid, and assets have to be conserved. If no durable power of attorney is in place, legal action through the court will be necessary before anyone can act on the patient's behalf. There are basically two legal approaches to assisting and protecting the patient: a conservatorship or limited guardianship.

GUARDIANSHIP/CONSERVATORSHIP VERSUS LIMITED GUARDIANSHIP

The differences between guardianship/conservatorship and limited guardianship are defined by state laws. In general the conservator handles the property, including real estate, personal property, and money. The court may also appoint a guardian or conservator to have charge and custody of the patient. This much control may not be necessary in all cases. Under such circumstances the limited guardianship program may be employed. A limited guardian has only the responsibilities defined by the court.

Public Guardianship

A few states have established public guardianship programs. The public guardian provides for a disabled person's needs when no responsible family members or friends are willing or available to serve as guardian. This program is also appropriate if the disabled person cannot afford the services of a private guardian.

The actions of a public guardian, of all guardians and conservators, are supervised by the courts. For example, approval has to be obtained before real estate, cars, or furniture can be sold. Court approval is also required for major purchases. Once a year an accounting is made to the court listing all income and expenditures. Bills and cancelled checks are also presented to the court. The overall rule is that the guardian must manage the financial affairs of the disabled person in the manner of a prudent person at all times.

In addition to the financial assets, if the conservator or guardian has charge of the person, there are other responsibilities, which may include ensuring that the patient is adequately housed, fed, and clothed and that he receives regular medical care. At all times the guardian has the responsibility to encourage the ward to take part in decisions whenever possible.

Another duty often placed on a conservator or guardian is to give informed consent for the care and medical treatment of the disabled person. It is important to note that the relative who signs the forms as the responsible party when the patient is admitted to the hospital or nursing home does not automatically have the legal authority to make decisions or to authorize treatment for a patient. The responsible party is only responsible for paying the bill. It is the guardian or conservator of the person or the limited guardian who has been given the specific authority over health care decisions who can authorize treatment. The conservator or guardian makes the health care decisions for the disabled person, decisions that would normally be made by a competent patient.

In most states it is not necessary to prove the patient legally incompetent before the court appoints a conservator or guardian. The law requires only that the person be mentally and/or physically disabled or incapacitated and thus unable to handle his own affairs. Proper notice, medical evidence, and a hearing in court are required. The court decides whether the appointment is needed and appropriate. The appointed guardian or conservator must be someone the court finds both willing and capable of serving in that capacity.

Sometimes there may be a person who is very willing to serve but who has ulterior motives. For example, one woman's grandson moved in with her. He brought along his wife and three teenage children. They had no income. Everyone in the house lived on the woman's Social Security check. The grandson spent all of his grandmother's savings. He cashed in her certificates of deposit and then sold some of her furniture. Outraged neighbors contacted Adult Protective Services at the Department of Human Services, and the agency stepped in to protect the grandmother. Needless to say, the judge felt that the grandson might be willing to serve, but he did not appoint him as conservator.

Often a willing relative may be too frail and disabled to handle the job. In other cases relatives simply do not want to take the responsibility. If there is no money to hire an attorney or a trust department at a bank, the public guardian may be appointed.

Procedures in establishing a conservatorship or limited guardianship are fairly similar. For a patient with Alzheimer's disease, the petition is most likely to be for a full guardianship or full conservatorship, since the patient may eventually be unable to handle any of his affairs. The first step in establishing a guardianship or conservatorship requires a petition to be drawn up by an attorney and then filed with the Chancery Court. The request for a petition can be made by the disabled person himself, by a family member, or by any other concerned person. Sometimes the Department of Human Services petitions the court. Hospital or nursing home administrators may petition the court when they realize the need for such an appointment.

Once the petition is filed, a date is set for the hearing. Most states specify the number of days' notice that must be given to the person for whom a guardian or conservator is to be appointed. Notice is also given to the spouse, children, or next of kin, unless the person files the petition himself. The notice is sent by registered mail or served by a sheriff's deputy.

Before the court hearing (which can be delayed up to 60 days), the court appoints a guardian ad litem to serve for this one action only. The role of the guardian ad litem is to protect the interests of the person being considered for a guardianship or conservatorship. The guardian ad litem completes a thorough study of the patient's situation. At the hearing, she represents the person by questioning the witnesses and the potential conservator.

The court may subpoena witnesses, such as nurses who have cared for the patient, a neighbor, or anyone who has been involved in the case. The law may require the testimony of at least two physicians, which may be submitted in a written document, by deposition, or in person. The judge decides at the hearing if a guardian or conservator is needed. If such a finding is made, the judge then appoints the guardian or conservator.

After the appointment has been made, all costs are paid out of the disabled person's funds. This includes the petitioning attorney's fee, the fee of the guardian ad litem, and the court costs. The procedure is not inexpensive. If the court decides that the appointment of a guardian or conservator is not appropriate, the person who filed the petition must pay the fees and costs.

A number of difficult choices face the guardian or conservator. The question of when it is best to transfer assets of the patient with Alzheimer's disease is a very difficult one to answer. As the patient's assets decline, he may become eligible for Supplemental Security Income (SSI) and/or Medicaid. Therefore, the laws and regulations governing these benefits must be considered before assets are transferred. Currently Medicaid regulations do not require applicants to sell their homes before receiving benefits. To retain the home the only requirement is that hospital or nursing home patients express their desire or intention to return to their home. A written statement to this effect can even be made on behalf of a comatose patient. An "intent to return home statement" results in having the home excluded from the countable assets of a Medicaid or SSI applicant. In some states assets in the patient's name, other than the home, that exceed a specific amount must be used for the care of a patient in a nursing home before Medicaid eligibility is established. For example, in 1989 a single resident in the state of Tennessee could keep up to $2,000 in countable assets while receiving Medicaid benefits.

Any transfer of assets occurring within 2 years before the application for Medicaid initiates an official audit. Transfer of assets at less than fair market value during that 2-year period creates a presumption that the person is trying to fraudulently establish Medicaid eligibility. For example, selling the patient's $6,000 car to a son for $200 could lead to a disqualification for Medicaid. Most states have a law making it a felony to transfer property for the purpose of obtaining or keeping Medicaid eligibility.

If a transfer of assets is not made early in the illness, the possibility of needing Medicaid in the future should be considered before any transfers are made. If Medicaid application is even a remote possibility, a consultation with someone well schooled in the requirements of this program is suggested.

In summary, immediate financial and legal planning is necessary as soon as Alzheimer's disease is diagnosed or strongly suspected. These plans should be developed under the guidance of an attorney. Appropriate steps taken during the early stages of the disease will enable the caregiver, family member, or appointed guardian to protect and make the best use of all assets during the remaining lifetime of the patient with Alzheimer's disease.

BIBLIOGRAPHY

Overman W Jr and Stoudemire A: Guidelines for legal and financial counseling of Alzheimer's disease patients and their families, Am J Psychiatry 145(12):1495-1500, 1988.

UNIT SIX
TECHNICAL ASPECTS

22

The aging process

R. Hamdy

Despite all of modern medicine's technical, and scientific advances, the maximum life span of human beings has not increased significantly since ancient times. Indeed, there is evidence that in ancient Roman times a few people lived to the age of 100 years. Even before then, during ancient Egyptian times, records indicate that some people also reached old age. For instance, it is documented that one of the Egyptian pharaohs, Ramses II, lived to the age of 92 years. At that time, should a pharaoh show signs of mental incompetence, it was customary to assume that "evil forces" had taken over his mind and to perform a trephine operation to let the "evil spirit" out. A trephine operation consisted of drilling a hole through the skull bone. This was in most instances a fatal intervention for the pharaoh and a "sad incidental happening," but it provided a practical solution to the problem of having an absolute monarch whose impaired mental functions could jeopardize the future of the nation. It can be assumed, therefore, since Ramses II was still governing Egypt by the age of 92, that he was mentally competent. Indeed history indicates that his reign was one of the most successful.

Reaching very old age, therefore, was not unknown in antiquity. Yet, even nowadays relatively few people survive past the age of 100 years, and reaching that age is still regarded, at least in some countries, as a remarkable achievement. In the United States, for instance, the person who reaches 100 years receives a congratulatory telegram from the president on his or her birthday.

The main change modern science and medicine have brought to our civilization is an increase in the life expectancy of the individual. The main difference in the population living now in the late 20th century in the Western hemisphere compared with the population living in ancient

Roman or Egyptian times (or with the population living earlier this century in the Western hemisphere) is that currently many more people reach an old age and achieve their maximum life potential. In fact the main difference between the survival curve of ancient Rome and that of the United States in the 1980s is that currently fewer people die at a young age in the United States and therefore many more people live longer. In other words, the life expectancy has increased even though the life span has remained essentially unchanged.

It may be of interest also to note that the main change has occurred during this century. The survival curve of the population living in the Unites States in the earlier years of this century is not too different from that of the population living in ancient Rome. Modern science has not succeeded in significantly prolonging the human life span, but it has succeeded in preventing people from dying at an early age, thereby allowing a larger proportion of the population to reach old age. In the United States the life expectancy at birth has risen from 47.3 years in 1900 to 74.5 years in 1982.

This increased life expectancy is mostly the result of the control and successful treatment of acute illnesses. Diseases such as pneumonia, tuberculosis, and plague, which used to be almost uniformly fatal a few decades ago, currently are very easily treated. It is a sobering thought that antibiotics did not become commercially available until after the Second World War. Until that time physicians had no effective means of helping patients overcome infections that were often fatal.

Currently, in Western civilization, relatively few people die in early youth, and if they do it usually is either the result of violence, accidents, or in rare cases a fatal disease. Unfortunately, there are still a few genetic, malignant, and rare diseases that are lethal to young people. Sadly, in these times a number of deaths in young adults are attributed to acquired immunodeficiency syndrome, or AIDS. On the whole, however, death among young people in our society is so unexpected it is regarded as very unusual or "shocking."

DISEASES COMMON IN OLD AGE
Chronic Degenerative Diseases

Although many of the acute fatal illnesses have been largely controlled, they have been replaced by chronic illnesses that are mostly degenerative in nature and that usually have an insidious onset and a slow rate of progress. Not infrequently they are erroneously considered part of the aging process. This often leads the patient to delay seeking medical advice until the condition is well advanced and the scope for successful treatment is limited.

Multiple Pathologies and Polypharmacy

The presence of more than one illness at the same time means that the patient is likely to be prescribed a number of medications, often by different physicians, for long periods. Not infrequently, the patient who does not see any satisfactory improvement will seek the advice of more than one physician, often without telling each physician that he is already under the care of another physician or has been seen by other physicians, who have prescribed some medication that he is still taking. The two major health problems of old age are multiple pathologies and polypharmacy. Often the latter aggravates the former, and a vicious circle sets in, when more medication is prescribed to control the side effects induced by a medication prescribed earlier.

NO MEDICATION IS FREE OF SIDE EFFECTS

I had a patient who illustrates this point well. Mrs. S. was in her early sixties, in good mental and physical health, and taking no medication. Her husband had just retired, and since both were keen badminton players, they had started playing more frequently and for longer periods. She developed pain in her knees and went to see her physician, who diagnosed "early osteoarthritis" and prescribed an analgesic/antiinflammatory medication. This seemed to help Mrs. S; the pain was relieved, and she was able to play for longer periods and more frequently.

Gradually, however, she noticed that she tended to become breathless and that at the end of the day her legs often became swollen. At first she did not pay much attention to this, but when her breathlessness interfered with her ability to play badminton, she consulted her physician again. He diagnosed "congestive cardiac failure" and prescribed three more drugs: digoxin, to improve the efficiency of the heart; diuretics, to increase the volume of urine produced and reduce the work load on the heart; and potassium supplements, to compensate for any potassium loss induced by the diuretics. Mrs. S. was now taking four different medications. Her breathlessness improved significantly and the swelling of her legs had almost completely disappeared.

However, she became aware of another problem: She was producing large quantities of urine soon after taking her diuretic. Initially, this interfered with her badminton game, but she soon discovered that she could get around this problem by taking the diuretic tablet after rather than before the game. As time went by, however, she experienced difficulties in holding her urine long enough to reach a restroom and had a few accidents in which she wet herself. She consulted her physician once again; he explained that because of her advancing age, the capacity of her urinary bladder was gradually decreasing, and taking diuretics, which increase the urine volume, did not help much. He nevertheless prescribed oxybutynin, a drug meant to increase the capacity of the bladder. Mrs. S. was now taking five different drugs.

As time went by, although her breathlessness during the day had improved, she experienced severe bouts of shortness of breath at night, bouts that frequently woke her up. She again consulted her physician, who explained that this was most probably the result of her heart failure and prescribed three more drugs; salbutamol and aminophylline to dilate the tracheobronchial tree (airways) and a sleeping tablet to allow her to sleep well at night. Mrs. S. was now taking eight different drugs. Since she was motivated and anxious to get better, she took these tablets regularly, although her husband often had to remind her to take them.

As more time went by, although Mrs. S. was by-and-large asymptomatic (she had no pain in her knees, was not short of breath, had no swelling in her legs and slept well at night), she nevertheless appeared to have become apathetic and lethargic and to have lost interest in virtually everything. She did not feel like playing badminton and spent most of her time lying in bed. Not infrequently she did not even bother to get dressed. Her husband became worried and insisted that she visit her physician again. At the end of the consultation, the physician felt that Mrs. S. was depressed and prescribed an antidepressant and some vitamin tablets. She was now taking 10 different medications.

A few days after visiting her physician and despite taking her medication regularly, she became short of breath and developed a productive cough and fever. Her husband took her to her physician, who arranged for her to be hospitalized.

In the hospital a diagnosis of pneumonia was made, and the appropriate medication was prescribed. A few days later Mrs. S.'s pneumonia was controlled, she was discharged, and was followed up in the outpatient clinic. The physicians there, suspecting that many of her problems were related to medication, gradually stopped the medications she had been taking. About 12 weeks later she was taking no medication, feeling much better, and even started playing badminton again, taking only the occasional pain-killer when her knee became painful.

Mrs. S.'s case illustrates an important point, that often a medication is prescribed to counteract a side effect of another medication previously prescribed. In Mrs. S.'s case the analgesic/antiinflammatory medication initially prescribed precipitated heart failure, the diuretic induced urinary incontinence, and the sleeping tablets made her weak, lethargic, and seemingly depressed. None of these symptoms were related to her age; her condition improved dramatically once all the medications were stopped.

AVOIDING POLYPHARMACY

Polypharmacy can be avoided by insisting that patients bring all the medication they have in the house, including those purchased over the counter, to the physician. Because medication is so expensive, patients often hoard it against the day when it "may be needed again." The physician can then decide whether the patient's current condition could be the result of some side effect of the medication or whether it is caused by a disease that needs another medication. Furthermore, if the physician knows the medications the patient is already taking, she is not likely to prescribe one that may interact and interfere with those medications.

DISEASES ARE NOT PART OF THE NORMAL AGING PROCESS

It is interesting to note that many of the diseases that afflict older people have been known since antiquity. It is important to realize that although many ailments such as repeated falls, urinary incontinence, and impotence are often seen in old age, they by no means constitute an integral part of the aging process. It must be stressed that a person can age and yet enjoy good health in the same way as another person can be in poor health and young. Old age is not necessarily associated with disease and poor health.

A look around shows that many people in very prominent places are over 65 years of age. Whether they are in the political, scientific, industrial, financial, legal, or artistic field, they occupy important positions and are still very active mentally and/or physically. In many respects their capabilities far exceed those of the younger generation.

THE "NORMAL AGING PROCESS" IS DIFFICULT TO STUDY

The study of the aging process is a very difficult field because of all the diseases that are frequently found in old age. The difficulty lies in differentiating processes associated with normal aging from those associated with diseases commonly seen in old age. This is one of the reasons why a number of cross-sectional studies have yielded inaccurate and misleading results about the aging process.

For instance, it used to be generally accepted that the aging process was associated with a gradual decline in the functions of most of the body organs. This belief was based largely on a number of cross-sectional studies of various people in different age groups, calculating the average (mean) results of the parameters studied and observing that the mean tended to drop as older people were studied. Since the late 1950s, however, a number of longitudinal studies have been set up and are still in progress. The preliminary results indicate two important facts: Not everyone ages in the same way or at the same rate, and there is a large degree of interorgan variability. There is also a growing body of evidence that some individuals may age without any deterioration in their body functions.

FACTORS THAT MAY AFFECT THE FUNCTIONS OF AGING ORGANS

Even when the same population is followed for a number of years, the study of aging can be quite controversial for a number of reasons. First, it is very difficult to define what is "normal." For instance, if only a population completely free of disease is considered, is this a "supernormal" population (the biological elite) or are these simply normal individuals who have been lucky to escape disease? If this is a supernormal population, can it then be compared to other people of a different age group? Shouldn't "supernormal" individuals in all age groups be studied?

Second, even if the aging process is associated with a decline in various body functions, quite a number of factors affect the rate of this decline. Not infrequently these factors are independent of the particular organs studied. For instance, a person with osteoarthritis of the knees or hips who has been taking analgesics or nonsteroidal antiinflammatory medication for a number of years may have worsened renal functions, because this medication often leads to deterioration of the kidney functions. In this case the renal functions would be worse in this person than in another of the same age and sex, even though that person had not had any renal disease. Similarly, a number of diseases may interfere with the functions of various body organs. Many of these diseases are often seen in older patients, and they may have induced changes that may be erroneously attributed to the aging process.

EFFECT OF AGING ON MENTAL FUNCTIONS

A number of factors affect a person's intellectual capabilities, particularly the person's education and the degree of mental stimulation that he enjoys. It also must be emphasized that the education the average person receives nowadays at school and college is much more technical than the one a person would have received 50 or 60 years ago. Many things that are now a part of our daily life such as computers, word processors, and television did not exist 50 or 60 years ago. It would be both unfair and erroneous to compare the problem-solving ability of older people today (who were at school and college more than 60 years ago) with young people just out of college.

Furthermore, if the same population is followed longitudinally, the rate of change in intellectual and mental capabilities depends on the degree of mental stimulation the person receives. Indeed, unless they are afflicted by some disease, professionals who continue to work and be involved in their field of interest seldom show signs of decline in their specialty, even though they may get out of touch with developments in other fields. Unfortunately, a number of people on reaching the age of retirement drastically reduce their degree of mental stimulation. This often leads to a rapid decline in intellectual capability, in a way similar to the athlete who stops training and becomes physically deconditioned. Mental stimulation maintains the mental functions in the same way that physical stimulation maintains physical fitness.

Finally, as has already been emphasized earlier in this chapter, a number of medications can affect a person's intellectual capability. These include in particular the sedative and hypnotic preparations. Other medicines also may have similar effects, such as drugs used to reduce blood pressure and even some cold remedies.

It is also important to appreciate that many drugs persist for a much longer period in older people than they do in younger ones. Sedative and hypnotic drugs may have a much longer duration of action in older people.

It is felt that by now, readers will appreciate some of the difficulties involved in researching the aging process and the need to carefully examine the methodology of various studies before interpreting the results. In the light of these comments, it might now seem appropriate to concentrate on the effects of aging on the central nervous system.

AGING AND THE CENTRAL NERVOUS SYSTEM

The total weight of the brain and its size have been reported to decrease in old age; the average loss being 7% to 8% from the peak weight reached in adulthood. It must be emphasized, nevertheless, that these are the results of cross-sectional studies (and therefore subject to a number of factors not necessarily related to the aging process). It is interesting to note that in some instances, young adults were found to have brain weights lower than those of older people.

Although both the gray and white matter of the brain show some loss and atrophy, it has been postulated that more gray matter is lost in the early decades (20 to 50 years) and more white matter is lost in the later ones. An age-related increase in the size of the ventricles also has been reported, specially after 60 years of age.

The loss of brain weight is associated with narrowing of the gyri and atrophy of the cortical sulci. There is also evidence that the reduction in the number of nerve cells does not affect the brain uniformly, but tends to be particularly pronounced in some areas.

It has been suggested recently that the degree of age-related neuronal loss is only minimal, but that the neuronal size tends to decrease with age and that this decrease in size of the nerve cells is responsible for the smaller size of the brain and its reduced weight. In Alzheimer's disease, on the other hand, neurons actually die.

Some specific microscopic changes have been observed in the aging brain, particularly after the fifth decade. These include the appearance of neurofibrillary tangles, senile plaques, granulovacuolar degeneration, and the accumulation of "age" pigments (lipofuscin, ceroid, and neuromelanin). In Alzheimer's disease, these changes are much more pronounced.

It has been suggested that the cerebral blood flow may decrease in old age. However, there is no sufficient evidence that in the absence of disease, either the cerebral blood flow or the cerebral oxygen utilization are affected by the aging process. Aging does not appear to interfere with the overall functions of the brain. Reduction in intellectual capabilities are, therefore, secondary to diseases or to social and psychological factors not necessarily related to the aging process.

AGING AND IMPAIRED VISION AND AUDITORY ACUITY

It is important to realize that elderly people often have reduced visual and auditory acuity. It has been estimated that about 1.4 million people in the United States suffer from severe visual impairment. Of these approximately 990,000 are over 65 years of age. The three main diseases responsible for diminished vision are glaucoma, cataracts, and senile macular degeneration of the retina. In addition, the curvature of the cornea becomes less smooth and more irregular in old age (a condition known as astigmatism), and frequently light entering the eye may be refracted by deposits in the cornea, which are increasingly present in old age.

Although many elderly people wear eyeglasses, these are frequently inadequate. It is recommended that older people have their eyeglasses checked at regular intervals of 2 or 3 years or whenever their eyesight seems to have deteriorated. It is also a sad but frequent sight to find many people in nursing homes or other institutions wearing glasses that are covered with a layer of dust, further interfering with the patient's visual acuity. It should be the responsibility of the caregivers, attendants, and supervisors to ensure that the patient's glasses are kept clean.

Impaired hearing acuity may prevent the patient from taking part in a sensible conversation. Furthermore, the distortion of sounds heard may lead the patient to misinterpret the question and give an inappropriate answer. It is important before assessing the patient's mental functions to make sure that he can hear adequately and that there is no significant hearing loss, or the results of the tests may be false.

OLDER PEOPLE AND ISOLATION

People with visual or auditory impairment often find themselves mentally isolated from the rest of society, and they find it increasingly difficult to cope with the high technology demands made by various gadgets often used in everyday life. This tends to make the elderly withdraw from society.

The often associated diseases present in old age tend to make the elderly also gradually withdraw from physical activity. Osteoarthritis makes movements of the joints painful, Parkinson's disease makes the movement difficult. Unless the older person has been exercising, the decreased respiratory and cardiac reserve capacity would make him become short of breath much quicker than younger people. As a result of all these handicaps, older people often tend to gradually isolate themselves physically and tend to lead a more sedentary life.

Last but not least, because most elderly people have a fixed income, they often are reluctant to use their limited funds to engage in activities that would increase their socialization.

Because of a combination of mental, physical, and financial isolation, elderly people often become so cut off from the rest of society that their circle of friends and acquaintances gradually shrinks, until their only contact is their spouse. At this stage it can be easily understood what happens when the spouse either becomes ill, is affected by a condition such as Alzheimer's disease, or dies.

It must be emphasized, nevertheless, that despite all these handicaps, elderly people can maintain a high level of intellectual involvement and that mental impairment is not an integral part of the aging process.

BIBLIOGRAPHY

Arnetz BB: Interaction of biomedical and psychosocial factors in research on aging: a European perspective, Ann Rev Gerontol Geriatr 5:56-94, 1985.

Barnes CA: Aging and the physiology of spatial memory, Neurobiol Aging 9(5-6):563-568, 1988.

Black JE et al: Environment and the aging brain, Can J Psychol 41(2):111-130, 1987.

Brayne C and Calloway P: Normal ageing, impaired cognitive function, and senile dementia of the Alzheimer's type: a continuum? Lancet 1(8597):1265-1267, 1988.

Burchinsky SG: Neurotransmitter receptors in the central nervous system and aging: pharmacological aspect (review), Exp Gerontol 19(4):227-239, 1984.

Drayer BP: Imaging of the aging brain. I. Normal findings. II. Pathological conditions, Radiology 166(3):785-796, 797-806, 1988.

Emery OB: Language and aging, Exp Aging Res 11(1):3-60, 1985.

Featherman DL and Petersen T: Markers of aging. Modeling the clocks that time us, Res Aging 8(3):339-365, 1986.

Feinson MC: Aging and mental health. Distinguishing myth from reality, Res Aging 7(2):155-174, 1985.

Fitzgerald DC: The aging ear, Am Fam Physician 31(2):225-232, 1985.

Hamill RW et al: Neurodegenerative disorders and aging. Alzheimer's disease and Parkinson's disease—common ground, Ann NY Acad Sci 515:411-420, 1988.

Hayflick L: Theories of biological aging, Exp Gerontol 20(3-4):145-159, 1985.

Hoenders HJ and Bloemendal H: Lens proteins and aging, J Gerontol 38(3):278-286, 1983.

Leaf A: The aging process: lessons from observations in man, Nutr Rev 46(2):40-44, 1988.

Long DM: Aging in the nervous system, Neurosurgery 17(2):348-354, 1985.

Masoro EJ: Physiological system markers of aging, Exp Gerontol 23(4-5):391-397, 1988.

McGeer PL: The 12th J. A. F. Stevenson memorial lecture. Aging, Alzheimer's disease, and the cholinergic system, Can J Physiol Pharmacol 62(7):741-754, 1984.

Moran MG and Thompson TL II: Changes in the aging brain as they affect psychotropics: a review, Int J Psychiatry Med 18(2):137-144, 1988.

Morse DR: Aging: causes and control, Int J Psychosom 35(1-4):12-42, 1988.

Pedley TA and Miller JA: Clinical neurophysiology of aging and dementia, Adv Neurol 38:31-49, 1983.

Pepeu G: Acetylcholine and brain aging, Pharmacol Res Commun 20(2):91-97, 1988.

Price DL et al: Neurobiological studies of transmitter systems in aging and in Alzheimer-type dementia, Ann NY Acad Sci 457:35-51, 1985.

Reuben DB, Silliman RA, and Traines M: The aging driver. Medicine, policy, and ethics, J Am Geriatr Soc 36(12):1135-1142, 1988.

Roth GS and Joseph JA: Peculiarities of the effect of hormones and transmitters during aging: modulation of changes in dopaminergic action, Gerontology 34(1-2):22-28, 1988.

Scott RB and Mitchell MC: Aging, alcohol, and the liver, J Am Geriatr Soc 36(3):255-265, 1988.

Speech understanding and aging. Working Group on Speech Understanding and Aging. Committee on Hearing, Bioacoustics, and Biomechanics, Commission on Behavioral and Social Sciences and Education, National Academy of Sciences–National Research Council. J Acoust Soc Am 83(3):859-895, 1988.

Straatsma BR et al: Aging-related cataract: laboratory investigation and clinical management, Ann Intern Med 102(1):82-92, 1985.

Veith RC and Raskind MA: The neurobiology of aging: does it predispose to depression? Neurobiol Aging 9(1):101-117, 1988.

Vernadakis A: The aging brain, Clin Geriatr Med 1(1):61-94, 1985.

Walsh DA: Aging and visual information processing: potential implications for everyday seeing. Part I. J Am Optom Assoc 59(4):301-306, 1988.

Wisniewski HM and Wen GY: Lipopigment in the aging brain, Am J Med Genet 5(suppl):183-191, 1988.

23

The normal brain: an overview

P. Sloan

Humans have known for centuries that the brain is the primary organ of thought and emotion. Scientists have discovered that the brain grows to weigh about 3 pounds by age 30 and then begins slowly to shrink. By using the brain's capacity for planning, problem solving, and communication, human beings have been able to travel to the moon, but much remains to be learned about how the brain actually works. Much of what is already known about the brain has come through the study of brain pathology. To better understand how a brain disorder such as Alzheimer's disease affects brain functioning, it is important first to have some basic understanding of the normal brain and its functions.

NERVE CELLS

The brain is made up of 140 billion cells, 20 billion of which are directly involved in processing information. Each of those cells has 15,000 direct physical connections with other brain cells. This is an organism that is far more complex and sophisticated than a main frame computer.

Nerve cells are made up of several different types of cells. Regardless of the type, each nerve cell, or neuron, has a body, a stem (axon), and connecting branches (dendrites). Neurons within the brain are interconnected and operate primarily on the basis of electrical and chemical activity. Through the combination of the two, a great amount of information is communicated among cells, both within certain areas and to distant parts of the brain.

The cell bodies give the brain a gray appearance on gross inspection; hence, the term "gray matter." The outer layer of the brain, which is called the cortex or neocortex, is made up mostly of cell bodies. The connecting nerve tissues are called glia cells. Because the axons of nerve cells bind easily to lipids (fat), they have a white appearance; hence the term "white matter." The white sheaths help speed conduction of nerve impulses. White tracks or fibers run from the outer layer of the cortex throughout the brain. Gray matter and white matter are terms used frequently when studying brain functioning.

BRAIN STRUCTURE

The brain is structurally divided into a left half and a right half, which are connected by a large bundle of white matter called the corpus callosum. The two halves are essentially symmetrical in appearance but not in function.

Scientists use various types of studies to examine brain structure and function. The comparative approach studies the brains of lower animals to learn comparatively about the structure and function of the human brain. Mammals are often studied because, like humans, they have a larger neocortex than lower animals. The cytoarchitectonic approach deals with the structure of cells, their differences, and how they are distributed throughout the brain. Some areas of the brain have cells that are six layers thick, whereas other areas may have only three layers of cells. These cells may be mapped to show differentiation in brain structure, which corresponds somewhat to brain function. The physiological method studies nerve structure, as well as electrical and biochemical activity of neurons. The study of electrical activities of nerve cells and how they are conducted has led to the development of instruments that produce recordings of brain function, such as the electroencephalogram (EEG) and evoked potentials (EP). As for the study of biochemicals, approximately 50 neurotransmitters have been discovered since 1950.

When a nerve cell is stimulated, an electrical impulse is generated and moves along the nerve cell. When the impulse reaches the end of the nerve cell, it stimulates the production and release of chemical compounds called neurotransmitters. One of these, acetylcholine, has been studied extensively in Alzheimer's disease. A deficiency in this neurotransmitter has been found in some patients with Alzheimer's disease. Acetylcholine is present in various parts of the brain and seems to have something to do with the laying down of memories in the cortex. Acetylcholine's precursor, choline, is contained in certain food substances such as lecithin that have been included in the diets of patients with Alzheimer's disease in hopes of improving memory. Unfortunately, these studies have not been too successful yet in terms of clinical treatment, although they have been most helpful in understanding neurochemical processes occurring in the brain.

Other neurotransmitters that have received much attention in the past couple of decades are dopamine, noradrenaline, serotonin, and enkephalins, or endorphins. Neurons that contain certain neurotransmitters appear to be organized in systems, and researchers try to relate these systems to particular brain functions. Chemicals in drugs that people take as medicine or for recreation can either increase or decrease the natural activity of these neurotransmitters, and much has been learned about how certain drugs affect behavior. Drugs that affect cognitive activity, "psychoactive" drugs, act on neurotransmitters in different ways, depending on the neurotransmitter system affected.

Stimulant drugs, such as amphetamines, release noradrenaline and block it reabsorption (reuptake) by the nerve cells. These drugs cause a general increase in arousal. Tricyclic antidepressants such as desipramine and imipramine block the reuptake of noradrenaline and serotonin, respectively, causing an antidepressant effect. Antipsychotic drugs such as chlorpromazine block the transmission of dopamine, creating a tranquilizing effect. Sedative hypnotic drugs such as alcohol, benzodiazepines, and barbituates reduce anxiety at low doses but produce sedation or coma at higher doses. These drugs decrease the activity of neurotransmitter systems that produce arousal, such as noradrenaline.

It should be noted that the neurotransmitter systems in normal elderly people may be more vulnerable to the effects of psychoactive drugs, possibly even more so if brain disease (e.g., dementia) has altered the normal number or activity of brain cells. Drug and neurotransmitter interactions can also cause a variety of complex reactions, which is why physicians use great care in prescribing psychoactive drugs for individuals suspected of having dementia.

Some neurotransmitters are made naturally within the brain. Endorphins, the natural tranquilizers and stimulants made within the brain, were discovered about 1975. These are thought to be generated by physical exercise—the "runner's high" that joggers speak of is probably the result of stimulation of these opiate-like substances. Acupuncturists believe that their needles stimulate endorphins, which act as natural anesthetics in some patients.

CENTRAL NERVOUS SYSTEM

The central nervous system is composed of the spinal cord and the brain. The neocortex, the outer covering of the brain, is the main focus of this discussion of higher brain (cortical) functions because it makes up about 80% of the human brain and separates humans from the lower animals. Only about 1.5 to 3 cm thick, the neocortex covers an area of up to 2,500 square centimeters. Nature folded and wrinkled the brain so that all of the surface would fit nicely into the human skull. Thus the brain has many ridges (gyri), grooves (fissures), and shallow grooves (sulci) that make up the cerebral cortex and give it its wrinkled appearance.

The brain and spinal cord are nourished by cerebrospinal fluid (CSF) that flows around the spinal cord and into the brain in a system of cavities called ventricles. In the normal brain the CSF is produced, circulates, and is reabsorbed freely. The ventricles can be viewed on a CT scan, a computer-generated X-ray picture of the brain. If brain tissue (neurons) has decreased, the ventricles may become enlarged to fill the space left by the loss of nerve cells. This shrinking of cortical matter is called cortical atrophy. Cortical atrophy and the resulting enlarged ventricles sometimes occur in individuals with dementia and can be clues in diagnosis.

HEMISPHERES AND LOBES

Structurally, the neocortex can be divided several ways. The simplest way, and the one most often used in the popular media, is to divide it into two halves, the left and the right cerebral hemispheres. Each hemisphere specializes in different functions, but typically they work in conjunction with one another. Whether the brain is considered as a whole or as two halves, it can be divided further into four basic divisions, or lobes. These lobes essentially are structural divisions at the deepest fissures. The frontal lobe constitutes basically the front, or anterior, half of the brain. In the back, or posterior, portion of the brain is the parietal lobe. The parietal lobe is evident on the outside, or lateral, surface and overlaps into the middle, or medial, surface of the cortex. The temporal lobe rests behind the temple, and the occipital lobe sits at the posterior pole above the cerebellum.

It is more complicated to try to divide the brain in terms of its functions, because it operates in an integrated fashion. Although certain neocortical regions or zones tend to specialize in certain brain functions, the brain works as an integrated functional unit. For example, individual instruments in a symphony orchestra and their functions may be described, but it is difficult to describe a particular piece of music being played by the orchestra as a function of individual instruments, because the composition is a functional whole. This is analogous to how the brain works.

BRAIN FUNCTIONS

One way of mapping brain functions is by stimulating the brain with tiny electrodes and recording what happens when certain parts of the brain are touched. This method has shown that in terms of primary motor and sensory function, the brain works largely in a contralateral fashion. This means that the side of the body that moves (motor function) or brings in information (sensory function) is on the opposite side of the half of the brain where this information is dealt with. To put it another way, the left half of the brain "controls" the right side of the body, and vice versa. It is not quite that simple, but for general purposes it can be thought of in that way. This is not to be confused with the popular notion of people being either "right brain" or "left brain" individuals, based on a predominance of specialized abilities. This notion refers more to complex higher cortical functions as related to thinking or personality style. Some people are thought to have better verbal skills (i.e., "left brain" functions) than visuospatial or artistic ones (i.e., "right brain" functions), or vice versa; hence the terms "left brain" and "right brain" people. The specialized abilities of each hemisphere are described later in the chapter. Basic sensory and motor functions are not addressed in detail; rather the focus is mainly on complex higher cortical functions.

Various models have evolved in the attempts to map and describe different brain functions. Over 200 years ago it was thought that certain brain functions could be localized to corresponding parts of the head. The "science" of phrenology tried to relate brain functions to the size of bumps on the head. Functions such as cautiousness, combativeness, benevolence, and language were thought to be located in certain areas. Phrenology became largely outdated by neuroanatomical research. ~~estingly~~, however, the language area was labeled as being next to ~~cause~~ the subject of study was a soldier who had received a ~~the~~ left eye and was unable to speak. In retrospect ~~t~~ the soldier's injury probably resulted in a lesion in ~~his~~ left frontal lobe, because Paul Broca, a French ~~vered~~ that this area controlled verbal output.

The advent in recent years of sophisticated radiological techniques have allowed brain functions to be studied in other ways. One of the most recent discoveries is Positron Emission Tomography (PET) wherein a person is injected with glucose containing radioisotopes. A computer-enhanced picture of the brain reveals in different colors areas of high and low glucose usage. The PET scan's predecessor, the CT scan, showed the structure of a person's brain. The PET scan reveals the actual brain functions in terms of what parts of the brain are active and inactive during certain types of mental activities such as thinking, speaking, looking, and listening.

Another way brain functions can be studied relatively inexpensively and without using extraordinarily sophisticated equipment is through the systematic study of cognitive and emotional behavior – the neuropsychological evaluation. Through the neuropsychological evaluation, what the brain actually does can be studied indirectly by examining what a person can and cannot do on various behavioral tasks (i.e., tests) of sensory, motor, and higher cortical functions, such as those of attention, concentration, memory, thinking, problem solving, and expression of emotions.

Generally speaking, the front part of the brain, the frontal lobe(s), has to do mostly with programming and execution of motor functions. At more complex levels of functioning, the frontal lobes orchestrate attention, thinking processes, planning, organizing, and abstract reasoning. The posterior part of the brain, the parietal lobe(s) has mostly to do with sensory perception. This involves taking in information from the environment. At more complex levels, the parietal lobes particularly have to do with the monitoring and organizing of all sensory input – visual, auditory, and tactile-kinesthetic. This makes sense geographically, because the parietal lobe lies between the temporal and the occipital lobe. The temporal lobe is responsible for audition, and the occipital lobe is primarily involved with vision. So, the parietal lobe is a conveniently located "switching station" for information. Thus the four basic lobes and their respective functions can be thought of as frontal with motor, parietal with sensory, temporal with audition, and occipital with vision.

To further describe the various levels of brain functions, the model developed by A.R. Luria will be used. Luria studied thousands of brain-damaged people and compared their brain functions to those of normal people. He divided levels of brain activity into functional units. These units are related to both areas, or zones, within the brain and to theoretical levels of functioning. Luria called these primary, secondary, and tertiary levels, or areas, of brain function. The primary level refers to immediate sensory and motor input and output. The secondary level relates to the association among or between the primary areas or zones. The tertiary level involves the zones that overlap and also has to do with higher levels of integration and organization of brain functions. Luria's model helps explain brain functions from the most simple to the most complex.

For example, consider the integration of various levels of brain function in the speaking of a heard word. First, a person must be awake at the basic level of arousal, a precursor to the activation of the primary projection areas of the brain. Projection refers to the actual recording or reception of sensory information. Once aroused, the temporal lobe is the primary projection area for audition. To repeat a word that has been heard, there first must be normal functioning of the auditory cortex in the left temporal lobe. After the sound is sensed, the signal is carried to Wernicke's area in the temporal-parietal area, where it is translated or decoded from a sound into a recognizable word. The passage of this signal and its translation involve the secondary area, or level of association. In turn, the message is carried forward by the white matter tracks to Broca's area in the frontal lobe. Broca's area translates or encodes the signal into its spoken form. Broca's area is directly adjacent to the motor strip, which controls the lips, tongue, vocal cords and palate so that the word can actually be verbalized. This communication among primary and secondary levels of the brain involves the tertiary level of complex brain functioning. That is, our actually thinking and recognizing what we are doing as we do it. The tertiary level also includes forethought and conscious appreciation of this process.

For a person to say a written word, the image is projected into the visual cortex of the occipital lobe. It is then carried forward into the association area of the parietal lobe and on forward to the motor speech area, which results in a verbal response. At first glance this seems to be a fairly simple, straight-forward process. These examples show that there is a relatively well-understood neurology for vision and for audition. However, the neurology for cognition, or complex thinking, is not yet quite as firmly established. These examples highlight how complex the actual processes are within and among various "functional units/levels" of the brain in the carrying out of complex behavior.

To discuss these higher cognitive processes, some of the other brain structures and their basic functions will be described and related to some of the more complex brain activities called higher cortical functions. For example, what processes are involved for someone to not only hear and see what is going on around them, but also to be simultaneously organizing the various events? This process includes understanding various perceptions and ideas congruently and planning the next action or some future action. For all of the motor, sensory, and associative processes to respond and act smoothly, the various brain functions must be working independently and in concert.

Cerebellum

The cerebellum sits under the cerebral hemispheres and facilitates the coordination and regulation of motor movements and, to some extent, cognitive activity. The cerebellum is an organ of synergy, whose functions can probably best be described by how they are negatively affected by alcohol. When a person has had too much alcohol, it interferes with the synergy of the cerebellum. That is why such a person has difficulty with gait and the coordination of smooth movements, such as touching the finger and nose in a rapidly alternating fashion. The cerebellum has far-reaching connections into the brain and spinal cord, predominantly coordinating the movement of independent parts of the body into a smoothly operating whole.

Reticular Formation

The reticular formation lies between the brain stem and the cortex and is responsible for activation, arousal, awakening, and paying attention. At a very basic level the reticular system deep in the brain has to be working to "turn on the light" in the cerebral cortex. For the brain to work normally, the cortex must be aroused by the reticular activating system in preparation for receiving and sending messages. This system both awakens the brain and keeps it "in tone" to receive sensory information and to execute motor and cognitive activity.

Cranial Nerves

The cranial nerves are special sensory and motor nerves arranged around the brainstem that communicate sensations and movements of the face, eyes, tongue, and vocal cords. They will not be described in detail; their specific location and functions can be reviewed in any good neurology text.

Basal Ganglia

The basal ganglia, which are made up of cell bodies, have a great deal to do with motor functions. They are symmetrically arranged and lie under the frontal cortex, with many connections to both the cortex above and the midbrain structures below. Loss of brain cells or neurochemicals in the basal ganglia and their connections can cause severe motor problems and, to a lesser extent, cognitive problems. Parkinson's disease, for example, affects nerve cells and neurochemicals in the basal ganglia, resulting in difficulties with posture, gait, and initiation and speed of motor activity.

The basal ganglia are also involved in the learning and programming of behavior. Activities that are repetitious and rehearsed over the course of life become somewhat automatic. For example, complex motor skills involved in walking, eating, or driving become so ingrained that a person does not have to think consciously to perform them. Some of these complex but well-programmed activities apparently are relegated to the basal ganglia. This may help explain why some of these complex behaviors are retained in people with dementia, sometimes long after severe loss of memory or language has occurred.

Thalamus

The thalamus is an important structure among the bundles of the basal ganglia that sit atop the brainstem. It is the central relay center for sensory and motor input and output. The thalamus must be working normally for all of the information coming in through the relay station to reach the cortex and then be relayed back to the spinal cord, which mediates the movement of the extremities. The thalamus is also involved in higher cortical functions, including memory and the coordination of complex acts involving various sensory input.

Limbic System

Needs, instincts, drives, and emotions are considered part of the functions of the deeper structures of the brain, the limbic system, or limbic lobe. It is called a system because its functions are thought to be related and to work together. Part of the limbic system, the amygdala, is instrumental in emotional functioning and is sometimes removed surgically in epileptics whose seizures are refractory to anticonvulsant medication. The hypothalamus is another part of the limbic system that rests deep within the brain and that generates drives such as hunger and sex. The hypothalamus also helps regulate other basic functions such as sleep, body temperature, emotions, and endocrine function. The pituitary gland, for example, which is very important to endocrine function, is located very close to the hypothalamus. Besides emotional and instinctual activities, the limbic system is also involved in cognitive activities. It is instrumental in both recording and generating memories.

INTEGRATION AND SPECIALIZATION OF HIGHER CORTICAL FUNCTIONS

In moving from the deeper brain structures and their functions to the cortex, complex cognitive functions called higher cortical functions are encountered. What processes are involved in logical thinking, association, memory, and problem solving, which are examples of higher cortical functions? There are many interconnections between the limbic system and the cortex, as well as within the cortex itself, and all of these connections contribute to the network of what is known as higher cortical functions. Much as with the instruments in an orchestra, all of the deeper and higher brain structures have to be both functional and working in concert for the tune (i.e., thought, behavior) to evolve as effective and synthesized.

By probing with electrodes the brains of people undergoing surgery, research has shown that different parts of the brain control different types of cognitive functions, as well as simple motor movements. Activities such as speech and the production of different types of verbal activity (e.g., nouns and verbs) are located in different brain areas. It has even been found, for example, that bilingual people control words differently and in different parts of their brain than do people who have only one language. The specialized functions of the brain have drawn popular interest in recent years, particularly since the fascinating split-brain experiments of Gazzaniga and his colleagues in the 1960s.

It is well known, for example, that most people are right-handed. As the brain tends to function contralaterally, it follows that language in most people is predominantly controlled by the left cerebral hemisphere. Research has shown that 99% of all right-handed people have language functions represented in the left cerebral hemisphere. That is why after a large stroke on the left side of the brain, patients often are paralyzed on the right side of the body and also tend to lose speech function. The left hemisphere is thought of as specialized for language and other special abilities relating to language, such as reading, listening to and remembering verbal material, and logical thinking. It is no surprise that because language is predominantly controlled by the left side of the brain, Broca's area is situated between the left temporal lobe, where verbal memories are generated and stored, and the motor strip, which controls the output of speech. Even in most left-handed people, who make up about 10% of the population, language is still "located" in the left cerebral hemisphere. Cases have been reported in which language was found to be distributed in both cerebral hemispheres, or predominantly managed by the right hemisphere. These cases usually resulted from familial (genetic) left-handedness or early developmental brain injury. More typically, however, the right hemisphere is thought to contribute to language functions less in direct or "linguistic" ways than through its involvement in attentional, organizational, or synthesizing activities.

The right cerebral hemisphere is typically more specialized for visuospatial functions involving a significant configural component, such as recognizing the parts of a puzzle as a whole picture, the ability to follow directions on a map, or the ability to look at a picture of a design and then build it from constructional materials. The right hemisphere is also thought to be more specialized for holistic, musical, and other nonverbal activities, such as recognizing and appreciating emotionality and solving problems or puzzles using nonverbal concepts. The right hemisphere functions have been described generally as more "creative" or "artistic" and the left hemisphere functions as more "logical" or "analytical."

Although the two hemispheres of the brain and other brain areas are specialized for certain functions, the entire cerebral cortex governs cognition (i.e., thinking and mental activity). The cerebral cortex is sometimes called the association cortex. The association cortex includes the frontal, parietal, temporal, and occipital lobes and other brain areas such as the cingulate gyrus and hippocampus of the limbic system, which are not directly involved in primary sensory and motor abilities. Although different brain regions are specialized for different activities, some functions are distributed throughout the brain. Memory is a prime example. For instance, the basal nucleus of Meynert, deep within the brain, is very much involved in generating mental activity and specifically has to do with the laying down of memories all over the cerebral cortex. Patients with Alzheimer's disease often have an unusually high number of neurofibrillary tangles and senile plaques in the basal nucleus of Meynert, such that these pathological cells and their related alterations in neurochemical activity interfere with the transmission of information into the higher levels of the brain. These examples show that the disruption of normal brain functions can be related to disease processes affecting specific brain areas and their connections. This is an extremely important concept in the study of diseases that cause abnormal behavior.

The parietal and frontal lobes seem to be especially important in complex higher cortical functions. The parietal lobes, for example, are the hub of sensory information and association. In fact, the inferior, or lower, portion of the left parietal lobe is believed to be the "association area of association areas." As was shown earlier, this brain area must be working normally for a person to speak and understand language or to read and write. The corresponding parietal lobe in the right cerebral hemisphere must be functioning normally for a person to accurately follow directions on a map, read a clock, and construct objects, such as in sewing a dress or building a birdhouse. The parietal lobes are also involved in organizing information and communicating it to the frontal lobes.

The frontal lobes constitute much of the area in the neocortex. The functions of the frontal neocortex are complex and least well understood and measured. It is known that the frontal lobes have much to do with the initiation and execution of motor behavior. They also are instrumental in the normal functioning of higher thought processes such as planning, abstract reasoning, trial-and-error learning, decision making, complex thinking, and problem solving. The frontal lobes also modulate intellectual insight, judgment, and the expression of emotions. A.R. Luria once described a farmer with frontal lobe damage as being in danger of starvation, not because the farmer would fail to eat from the cupboard for as long as there was food, but because he had lost his ability to plan ahead and initiate the planting of next year's crops and eventually would not replenish the cupboard and starve.

With this description of normal brain functions, it is easier to understand why patients with Alzheimer's disease have difficulty with cognitive functions. Early in Alzheimer's disease, a larger distribution of neurofibrillary tangles and senile plaques occur in the hippocampus and temporal and parietal lobes than in other brain areas. This disruption in normal brain functions early in the disease results in predominant impairment in memory, language, and constructional abilities. As the disease progresses, the frontal lobes and their connections may be affected. This can result in behavioral changes such as loss of initiative, spontaneity, and the ability to plan and organize behavior.

Perhaps, then, normal brain functioning and behavior can be defined as the condition when all of the brain's different structures and their functions are working properly, both independently and in concert. This is, of course, relative to the individual and his or her cultural surroundings. This definition is analogous to how normal intelligent behavior is defined, using such methods as intelligence tests and other neuropsychological instruments. David Wechsler, who developed the intelligence tests often used in assessing patients with suspected dementia, has said that the tests do not constitute intelligence per se. Rather, he said, they simply correlate with other, more widely accepted criteria of intelligent behavior. Thus the normal brain and its functions are defined in the context of the individual, his or her peer group, and the culture within which the person lives. Chapter 24 reviews the neuropsychological assessment of brain functions with regard to the evaluation of dementia.

BIBLIOGRAPHY

Bannister R: Brain's clinical neurology, New York, 1985, Oxford University Press.
Begley S, Carey J, and Sawhill R: How the brain works, Newsweek, pp 40-47, Feb 7, 1983.
Chusid JG: Correlative neuroanatomy and functional neurology, Los Altos, Calif, 1976, Lange Medical Publications.
Gazzaniga MS: The bisected brain, New York, 1970, Appleton-Century-Crofts.
Geschwind N: Disconnection syndromes in animals and man, Brain 88:237-294, 1965.
Geschwind N: Specializations of the human brain, Sci Am 241:180-199, 1979.
Heilman KM, Bowers D, and Valenstein E: Emotional disorders associated with neurological diseases. In Heilman KM and Valenstein E, editors: Clinical neuropsychology, New York, 1985, Oxford University Press.
Katzman RD: Alzheimer's disease, N Engl J Med 314:964-973, 1986.
Kolb B and Whishaw IQ: Fundamentals of human neuropsychology, San Francisco, 1980, WH Freeman & Co Publishers.
Lezak MD: Neuropsychological assessment, New York, 1985, Oxford University Press.
Luria AR: Higher cortical functions in man, New York, 1966, Basic Books.
Luria AR: The working brain, New York, 1973, Basic Books.
McKhann G et al: Clinical diagnosis of Alzheimer's disease, Neurology 34:939-944, 1984.
Snyder SH: Basic science of psychopharmacology. In Kaplan HI and Sadock BJ, editors: Comprehensive textbook of psychiatry, vol 4, Baltimore, 1985, Williams & Wilkins.
Wechsler D: The measurement and appraisal of adult intelligence, Baltimore, 1958, Williams & Wilkins.

24

Neuropsychological assessment of dementia

P. Sloan

This chapter focuses on the neuropsychological evaluation of brain dysfunction, particularly in dementia. The clinical neuropsychological evaluation attempts to describe both quantitatively and qualitatively the behavioral expression of brain dysfunction. This approach to assessment is historically rooted in clinical, physiological, and experimental psychology, behavioral neurology, and testing and measurement. Clinical neuropsychology has grown over the past several decades and is now a recognized subspecialty in most major medical centers and medium-sized communities. Most practicing neuropsychologists hold a doctor of philosophy in the behavioral sciences with additional predoctoral and/or postdoctoral training in the neurosciences. The goal of the evaluation is to measure and describe what the patient can and cannot do on various tasks of motor, sensory, cognitive, and emotional functioning; these findings are then correlated with activities of daily living (Sloan, 1984).

The typical evaluation attempts to address the following questions:
1. Is there evidence of brain dysfunction?
2. If so, is the degree of impairment mild, moderate, or severe?
3. Is there a particular pattern of impairment?
4. Are the degree and pattern consistent with a specific diagnosis such as a type of dementia?

The answers to these questions can shed some light on the course, prognosis, and management or treatment of the disorder and the effect it will have on the patient's caretakers.

Neuropsychologists use a variety of tests or a battery of tests (and tasks) to address these questions. The advantage to using standardized tests is that these tests typically meet scientific criteria of reliability and validity and thus can be replicated and interpreted among various neuropsychologists. The greatest statistical strength of most tests is their ability to distinguish between groups of patients with brain dysfunction of various types and degrees and those without brain impairment. Patients are also tested thoroughly in motor, sensory, cognitive, and emotional functioning, so that a battery of tests assesses a variety of brain functions in depth. This provides systematized observations of subtle cognitive and behavioral changes that may not be readily identifiable or quantifiable on a typical bedside physical, neurological, or psychiatric examination. This is especially true with regard to the measurement of the more complex higher cortical (brain) functions described in Chapter 23. Finally, because the tests record subtle or specific changes in mentation, they are well-suited for measuring such changes over time, an ideal approach in the study and management of progressive illnesses such as dementia.

PROCEDURES FOR CLINICAL NEUROPSYCHOLOGICAL EVALUATION

In theory, the neuropsychological measures attempt to "map" the various integrated, functional systems of the brain. To this end a typical battery includes a number of tests that may require a minimum of 3 hours of testing. Testing time can be longer with people who are less severely impaired. An evaluation costs about the same as a CT head scan. Except for patients who are in the very early stages of dementia, most patients suspected of having dementia cannot undergo several consecutive hours of testing because of cognitive impairment and fatigue. It has been more typical in my experience that patients, due to health, demographic, and cost factors, may be available for only one testing session limited to 3 hours or less. Thus the neuropsychologist must make good use of a selected number of measures that have been shown empirically to both reveal and distinguish dementia from other causes of brain dysfunction.

The typical evaluation incorporates available information from the medical, neurological and social history, combined with the usual clinical psychological procedures. These usual procedures include interviews with the patient, family, and/or associates; behavioral observations; and a mental status examination. Specific psychometric procedures are added to these routine procedures. The specific procedures may include an individually administered intelligence test and other standardized tests. These other tests cover attention, concentration, verbal and nonverbal memory, language, motor and somatosensory functions and specific higher order cognitive functions, such as complex reasoning, learning, and problem-solving skills.

Recent studies have shown that a number of brief cognitive screening instruments, such as the Modified Blessed Dementia Scale and the Mini Mental State Examination, are reliable in differentiating demented from nondemented individuals (Fillenbaum et al, 1987; Lesher and Whelihan, 1987). The Modified Blessed Dementia Scale, for example, has been correlated with neuropathological findings indicative of Alzheimer's disease (Katzman et al, 1983). Another brief checklist, the Hachinski Ischemic Score, has been shown to help differentiate Alzheimer's disease from multiinfarct dementia in patients with known histological diagnoses (Rosen et al, 1980). The use of these brief scales is but one example of the basic neuropsychological approach of quantitatively measuring cognitive impairment and empirically correlating such impairment with different types of dementia.

Neuropsychologists go beyond these basic screening measures to evaluate cognitive and emotional functioning more systematically and in depth. Most neuropsychologists use a group of tests designed to measure brain impairment. The particular tests or battery of tests usually reflect the individual neuropsychologist's training and experience but typically includes tests that have demonstrated empirical utility. Some of the best-known tests constitute or are selected from neuropsychological test batteries constructed by and named for reputable neuropsychologists and their colleagues such as Ward Halstead, Ralph Reitan, Arthur Benton, A.R. Luria, and others (Benton et al, 1983; Luria, 1966; Reitan and Wolfson, 1985). More recently developed batteries, such as the Luria-Nebraska (Golden, 1981), are still being researched and subject to controversy in the literature. Most practitioners have their own favorite tests and batteries and should be able to defend the use of their instruments on empirical and ethical grounds. Following are some tests and case examples from my experience that illustrate specific issues in neuropsychological assessment of dementia.

Nature of dementia

Although dementia is related to a number of causes, epidemiological studies indicate that the most common causes fall into a few categories, with Alzheimer's disease estimated to account for 50% to 60% of cases, multiinfarct dementia (MID) 10% to 15%, and a combination of the two (i.e., mixed) another 10% to 15%. The remaining small percentage is accounted for by other neurological disorders such as Huntington's disease, Parkinson's disease, progressive supranuclear palsy, AIDS dementia complex, and dementia associated with alcoholism (Fisk et al, 1983; Navia and Price, 1987). As for initial diagnosis, it is important to mention that it has been estimated that depression and other reversible medical problems may account for 10% to 30% of new cases. These so-called pseudodementias can be a complicating variable in initial assessment but are not necessarily progressive in themselves.

Fuld (1983) stated that the most frequent diagnostic differentiation posed to neuropsychologists is in evaluating for Alzheimer's disease versus multiinfarct dementia. Fuld's work is seminal for three reasons. First, she and her colleagues have successfully used neuropsychological tests to discriminate between groups of patients with dementia and normal elderly persons. Second, they have found different patterns of performance on these tests among different subtypes of dementia. Third, they have correlated these patterns with neuropathological findings and current theoretical understanding of dementing processes.

The Third Edition of the Diagnostic and Statistical Manual of the American Psychiatric Association-Revised (DSM-III-R) (American Psychiatric Association, 1987) lists the diagnostic criteria for dementia as demonstrable evidence of impairment in short- and long-term memory and impairment in at least one other area of higher cortical functioning. The latter category includes impairment in abstract thinking, judgment, or other disturbances such as aphasia (disorder of language), apraxia (inability to carry out motor activities despite intact comprehension and motor function), agnosia (failure to recognize or identify objects despite intact sensory functions), constructional difficulty (e.g., inability to copy designs), and personality change. To constitute a diagnosis of dementia, these impairments must interfere significantly with work, social, or interpersonal relationships.

Fuld (1983) and others (Katzman, 1986) have noted that Alzheimer's disease is characterized by large numbers of senile plaques and neurofibrillary tangles that usually appear early in the disease and are distributed more densely in the hippocampus deep inside the temporal lobes; later in the disease they are widespread throughout the cerebral cortex. Such patients have an associated deficiency in the cholinergic neurotransmitter system located in these respective brain areas. This probably helps explain why memory impairment is typically seen as an early, prominent sign of illness (i.e., hippocampal changes) followed by global intellectual decline with associated breakdown in other higher cortical functions (i.e., cortical changes). The most widely accepted current theoretical model of Alzheimer's disease explains specific behavioral changes on the basis of multiple, focal brain lesions that affect behavior in a predictable though heterogeneous manner, rather than as a diffuse, unpredictable process (Friedland et al 1988).

Multiinfarct dementia, on the other hand, is related to cerebrovascular disease and appears clinically when 50 to 100 g of brain tissue have been damaged (Fuld, 1983). The most common type of MID is the "lacunar state," which involves small lesions of the subcortical white matter and results in enlarged ventricles. The lacunar state does not seem to affect the cortex as much as other cases of MID. In "nonlacunar" MID, the cerebral gray matter is visibly damaged to the naked eye on autopsy. The latter type of MID causes small strokes at multiple cortical locations rather than the generalized cortical shrinkage seen in Alzheimer's disease. Also, the lacunar state type of MID does not result in as severe a picture of clinical dementia as does the other type of MID, Alzheimer's disease, or a combination of the two.

Clinical Differentiation

Neuropsychological tests have been useful in showing that patients with Alzheimer's disease perform more poorly on standardized tests than those with MID, who in turn perform more poorly than normal individuals (Fuld, 1983). Besides showing a greater degree of general cognitive impairment, patients with Alzheimer's disease differ from patients with MID on the tests in other characteristic ways. For example, although individual patients with Alzheimer's disease may perform somewhat differently from one another on the tests, their relative strengths and weaknesses typically remain consistent from initial diagnosis through the end-stages of the disease. That is, a patient with Alzheimer's disease who has predominant impairment in nonverbal memory and visuoconstructive ability but relatively good verbal skills will show these relative strengths and weaknesses over the course of the illness, regardless of how severe the impairment becomes. Patients with MID, on the other hand, show more variation in their test patterns from patient to patient and within the same patient over a period of time. This is presumably because of the more multifocal nature and "stuttering" course of MID (American Psychiatric Association, 1987).

In an ingenious series of studies, Fuld (1983) used some subtests of the Wechsler Adult Intelligence Scale (WAIS) to identify characteristic patterns of performance among various groups of demented and nondemented persons. Based on previous studies showing the cholinergic deficiency in patients with Alzheimer's disease, she found that a particular pattern of performance revealed in a previous study identified two consecutive groups of patients with Alzheimer's disease patients in another study. She derived this characteristic test pattern from the one found in a group of normal young adults with a temporary cholinergic deficiency induced by the drug scopolamine. The "Fuld profile" of the WAIS was highly specific for Alzheimer's disease among 138 consecutive referrals for dementia in that it produced only two false positives (two patients selected to have Alzheimer's disease who did not). Furthermore, although the profile interestingly resembles that expected in normal aging, the actual profile was found in less than 1% of 390 nondemented normal elderly people 75 to 85 years of age. Thus the profile is reasonably sensitive in that it allows identification of about 50% of all testable patients with Alzheimer's disease, but it is highly specific for the disease. The utility of the psychometric approach is further enhanced by the fact that the WAIS is such a commonly used and well-known IQ test, is both content and age appropriate for elderly persons, and is a thorough yet nonthreatening test for most patients. The following case illustrates the Fuld profile. The other case examples describe some of the more frequent diagnostic issues and other clinical considerations encountered in the neuropsychological assessment of dementia.

CASE STUDY 1: SENILE DEMENTIA OF THE ALZHEIMER'S TYPE (SDAT)

A 69-year-old, right-handed, retired professional man with an 18-month history of cognitive decline was referred as an outpatient for neuropsychological evaluation of dementia after an extensive medical evaluation proved unremarkable. There was no history of symptoms of cerebrovascular disease. Although his attention and concentration were adequate, he showed prominent memory loss for both recent and well-learned (i.e., remote) information. His WAIS scores revealed global intellectual decline (verbal IQ:94, performance IQ:82, full scale IQ:88) given his estimated premorbid level of above average to superior intellect (average IQ:90-100). Age-corrected scores on each of the selected WAIS subtests were consistent with the Fuld profile:

A = Vocabulary + information ÷ 2
B = Digit span + similarities ÷ 2
C = Digit symbol + block design ÷ 2
D = Object assembly
Fuld profile = A > B > C ≤ D; A > D

Interpretively, this tells us that this man's vocabulary and general fund of information were relatively well preserved, though still lower than expected for his educational and vocational experience. This is as expected, because these well-learned areas of knowledge are well retained and the last to deteriorate in either normal aging or dementing illness. His ability to recite strings of digits forward and backward (digit span) and his analysis of verbal similarities (e.g., How are an orange and banana alike?) were more impaired than his scores on the vocabulary and information subtests. The digit span and similarities subtests reflect auditory processing and immediate memory, and abstract reasoning, respectively. These more complex cognitive functions are more likely to deteriorate earlier in Alzheimer's disease. Similarly, the man's performance on timed tasks requiring visuospatial organization and visuomotor coordination and speed, the digit symbol substitution task and the visuoconstructive block design subtest, were even more impaired. Finally, his ability to construct puzzles of familiar objects (i.e., object assembly) was less impaired than the last two pairs of subtests but more impaired than the first pair, consistent with empirical data from Fuld's studies of patients with Alzheimer's disease. With the respective pairs of tests each represented by a letter, this man's age-corrected scores for the seven WAIS subtests corresponded to Fuld's profile (i.e., A > B > C ≤ D; A > D), which is suggestive of Alzheimer's disease.

This man also made one or more "intrusive" type perseverative errors, which have been found frequently among patients with dementia and are suspected to be characteristic of Alzheimer's disease in particular (Fuld et al 1982). These are errors in which the patient gives an inappropriate response to a question by carrying forward (i.e., "intruding") a response to a previous question even though other response(s) have occurred in between. For example, having given correctly the name of the current president earlier in the test, when asked, after several intervening questions, the name of a character in a brief story that had been read to him, the man answered again with the name of the president, which was grossly incorrect for the question asked.

The remainder of the neuropsychological tests revealed no particular pattern of sensorimotor or cognitive asymmetries suggestive of localized or lateralized brain dysfunction. That is, there were no findings suggestive of focal brain disease such as those found in patients with a stroke. Memory and other global intellectual impairments were prominent, and there were no significant motor findings suggestive of "subcortical" disease. The man's wife described personality changes of decreased spontaneity and initiative. The history and neuropsychological findings in this case were consistent with those of patients with Alzheimer's disease, which is the most definitive statement that can be made on the basis of the clinical neuropsychological evaluation, because Alzheimer's disease can be confirmed neuropathologically only on autopsy. Periodic re-evaluation, referral to the local Alzheimer's Disease Support Group, and consultation with the family were recommended.

CASE STUDY 2: MULTIINFARCT DEMENTIA (MID)

A 53-year-old, right-handed, disabled laborer with an eighth grade education was referred for neuropsychological evaluation of dementia upon admission to an inpatient psychiatry service. The patient was brought to the hospital by police officers, who reported that he was confused and had been rummaging in a large trash dumpster. His history included treatment for chronic hypertension and several episodes of suspected transient ischemic attacks (TIAs). On testing several days after admission, his orientation, attention, concentration and verbal memory (immediate, recent, and remote) were all commensurate with his education, despite his recent disorientation and confusion. Nonverbal recall for figures and visuoconstructive drawings were extremely impaired. The WAIS profile did not correspond to Fuld's profile for Alzheimer's disease and suggested instead mild global decline and specific impairment in functions served by the right cerebral hemisphere. Asymmetries were found on the sensorimotor examination, such as decreased index finger tapping speed on the left hand and impaired ability to recognize numbers written on the left fingertips (i.e., agraphesthesia). The Hachinski Ischemic Score (Hachinski et al 1975) was elevated and was positive for several markers suggestive of cerebrovascular disease such as abrupt onset, history of hypertension, stuttering course, and focal neurological symptoms. The clinical neuropsychological evaluation was strongly suggestive of right cerebral hemisphere dysfunction and MID, and thorough neurological evaluation for suspected stroke was recommended. Concurrent neurological examination, EEG, CT scan, and noninvasive blood flow studies suggested an infarct in the distribution of the right middle cerebral artery and bilateral carotid artery disease. The patient was treated accordingly and continued to improve until he reached a plateau in cognitive functions.

A pattern of multiple infarcts, either clearly identifiable or subtle, is typical of MID. These appear in a "patchy" distribution of deficits on the neuropsychological examination and tend to plateau after each event, each episode causing more dysfunction than the previous one. Typically, however, the course is one of a less severely progressive and rapid decline than in the typical patient with Alzheimer's disease unless a larger stroke occurs in the process. Yet, even when large strokes occur, unaffected areas of the brain often will be relatively functional. This picture is somewhat contrary to the global diminution in cortical function seen in Alzheimer's disease, particularly in the middle to late stages. In "mixed" cases having evidence of both Alzheimer's disease and MID, this distinction is more difficult to make.

CASE STUDIES 3 AND 4: SO-CALLED SUBCORTICAL DEMENTIAS

Case 3. A 73-year-old, right-handed woman was referred for evaluation of dementia as a medical inpatient after 48 hours of confusion and hallucinations possibly related to her medication (L-dopa for Parkinson's disease). She was alert and oriented, and she described her previous confusion, which was clearing. Her mental status examination revealed good attention, concentration, and recent recall, given her age and situation. Affect and personality were well preserved and bright despite marked difficulty with initiating motor and cognitive activity. Her face was masked, she was motorically rigid, and she could write only with great difficulty. As she was bedfast, extensive testing was impossible. Bedside examination revealed no significant impairment of language, motor praxis (the learned aspects of movements), calculation, or visuospatial perception, although she showed some mild impairment in complex cognitive functions and in drawing, writing, and movement. The movement impairment included the rigidity and micrographia (small handwriting) typical of Parkinson's disease. Although dementia could not be ruled out entirely by this evaluation, the "subcortical" motor impairment was far more prominent than any cortical cognitive manifestations, and the woman certainly did not appear likely to have Alzheimer's disease. This increased the possibility that her recent delirium was related to the suspected medication problem, which could be focused on further by her neurologist without undue concern about an interfering cortical dementia. She was referred for subsequent reevaluation as an outpatient but could not avail herself of the appointment because of her progressive Parkinson's disease.

Case 4. A 67-year-old, right-handed man with a professional degree was referred as a medical inpatient for evaluation of dementia because he answered most of the resident physician's questions with "I can't remember." Formal testing immediately revealed superb attention, concentration, and apparent cognitive awareness. When asked to recite a brief story read to him, however, he said, "I can't remember." When given a clue that the story was about a scrub-woman (the Anna Thompson story from the Wechsler Memory

Scale), he immediately recited most of the details of the story in chronological sequence. As he was clearly cooperative and did not appear significantly depressed, his difficulty in memory was revealed as one of difficulty in *initiating* recall, or retrieval, not one of registration and retention of information. The remainder of tests, including the WAIS, revealed relatively mild diminution of complex higher cortical functions; however, as with the woman in Case 3, severe impairment in motor functions was found. In this man impairment included significant slowing, stooped posture, rigidity, and oculomotor changes. The difficulties with eye movements were revealed by the neurologist to be typical of a subcortical disease affecting deep brain gray matter structures, a disease called progressive supranuclear palsy (PSNP). As a result of the neuropsychological evaluation, it was recommended that the patient be given verbal clues, or "boosts," to help him initiate action, both motor and cognitive, which helped significantly in his communication and self-esteem. As importantly, it was encouraged that he be socially stimulated and not be assumed to be more cortically impaired than he was, an unfortunately too frequent response to patients who are actually demented and sometimes to nondemented elderly persons as well.

Difficulty initiating and sustaining language, memory, and other cognitive activity, as well as motor activity, is typical of subcortical diseases. Although diseases such as PSNP, Parkinson's disease, and Huntington's disease usually include dementia as one of their complications, the cortical involvement usually occurs later in the disease process and is overshadowed by various motor symptoms early on. As the clinical neuropsychological evaluation includes both motor and cognitive tasks, relative quantification is useful in plotting the courses of such diseases, the response to medication, and the relative degree of motor versus cognitive impairment at various stages. Although there has been some controversy over the clinical distinction between cortical and "subcortical" dementias (Mayeux et al, 1983), neuropsychological test batteries carefully designed to quantify clinical differences have produced results that differentiate these dementia syndromes (Huber et al 1986).

CASE STUDY 5: THE AIDS DEMENTIA COMPLEX

A 28-year-old, right-handed clerk was referred as a medical inpatient for neuropsychological evaluation with a diagnosis of AIDS. The intern, who had treated a number of patients with AIDS, requested formal evaluation of cortical functions for what was described as "hazy" mentation. Navia, Jordan, and Price (1986) described a common disorder unique to patients with AIDS characterized by progressive dementia with accompanying motor and behavioral problems, which they termed the AIDS dementia complex. Consistent with recent literature (Navia and Price 1987), this young man's testing revealed mild to moderate global cognitive impairment. As with many patients with AIDS, this young man was mildly ataxic (had difficulty walking and with fine motor execution), dysarthric (had slurred speech) and "foggy" in attention, concentration, and mentation, but he had no outstanding or focal cognitive dysfunction.

Although the AIDS dementia complex usually develops after other complications of AIDS are evident, Navia and Price (1987) reported on 29 patients in whom progressive dementia with motor and behavioral disturbances were the first major signs of infections. As with many patients with AIDS who show only mild physical symptoms early in the illness, the dementia in this man was already apparent. Although somewhat reactively depressed, as expected, depression could not account for the degree of cognitive impairment found. This patient had characteristic difficulty with concentration and recent memory, mental slowing, and inability to perform complex activities of daily living such as finding his way around the hospital. Although the AIDS virus is known to attack the cerebral cortex directly, the effects of the disease are typically most apparent in the white matter and subcortical grey matter. This is the presumed reason that motor problems, particularly ataxia, leg weakness, and tremor, are often early signs in the complex, as with this patient. Clinically, the early cognitive and behavioral manifestations are more typical of the more subtle "subcortical" dementias than the cortical dementias; however, the AIDS dementia complex in its later stages can be nonsubtle in its destruction of the brain. The complex, with its cognitive, motor, and behavioral problems, can complicate severe cases of AIDS and appear either in isolation or as part of the AIDS-related complex with a variety of central nervous system complications. The course can be a rapidly deteriorating one to severe, bedridden dementia with mutism within a few weeks or months, or a milder, less precipitous course lasting many months to over a year.

This case also illustrates the importance of the evaluation of emotional functioning in the clinical neuropsychological examination. Although initially very stoical and denying of his illness, as rapport was established during interviewing and personality testing, the man's emotional lability became more apparent, and his concern about his illness, his family, and himself were expressed. While the testing established a good cognitive baseline against which future data could be compared, the evaluation also led to psychotherapeutic consultation with the patient, family, and staff. As his mentation deteriorated, assessment of emotional issues took prominence over cognitive measurement in assisting the patient and family.

CASE STUDY 6: ALCOHOL AMNESTIC DISORDER AND ASSOCIATED DEMENTIA

A 63-year-old, right-handed machinist was referred for neuropsychological evaluation as an inpatient on the intermediate medicine service, where he was still unable to walk, presumably because of peripheral neuropathy and ataxia following a brief stay on an acute medical ward for delirium. The medical evaluation was unremarkable and alcoholism and/or inadequate nutritional intake were denied by the patient. Careful review of the past medical record and interviews with relatives, however, revealed a strong likelihood of chronic and recent alcohol abuse and inadequate nutrition. Testing on consecutive days showed intermittent disorientation for time and place, as well as deficits in concentration, despite overall cognitive lucidity, facile conversational speech, and gregarious, shallow effect. There were no significant asymmetries on the sensorimotor examination, and complex higher cognitive functions showed only mild impairment, most apparent in visuoperceptual and visuomotor skills. Memory was grossly impaired, recent more so than remote, and the man frequently confabulated (i.e., filled in) missing details in memory. Except for poor memory, the test data suggested only mild global impairment; however, this patient frequently misidentified the examiner as being other familiar acquaintances and confabulated totally erroneous explanations of previous meetings, locations, and so forth. For example, he misconstrued a previous meeting on the acute medical ward as having occurred at a hospital in a distant state several weeks before the actual occurrence. He was inappropriately euphoric and nonchalant about his inaccuracies of memory and offered weak rationalizations. These behaviors were in striking contrast to his generally appropriate behavior on the ward and overall mildly impaired test performance.

All of these characteristics are fairly typical of the patient with alcohol amnestic disorder, or Korsakoff's syndrome. The disorder is relatively rare among chronic alcoholics as a unique entity in itself; however, the clinical distinctions among chronic substance abusers with varying degrees of dementia are not usually clear-cut, because difficulty in memory is frequently the most prominent dysfunction relative to other higher cortical functions. Korsakoff's syndrome is thought to be related to the deleterious effects of thiamine deficiency (and probably the alcohol itself) on deep-brain structures, whereas the milder forms of global dementia are associated with overall cortical deterioration. Yet it is most common to find on neuropsychological testing at least mild impairment in cognitive functions in chronic substance abusers, particularly in memory, visuoconstructive skills and visuomotor speed. It is not uncommon to see the clinical picture predominated by amnestic disorder features, whether or not a full-blown Korsakoff's syndrome is present. Similarly, in those patients who meet the diagnostic criteria for alcohol amnestic disorder, some degree of mild dementia is almost always present, as in the case previosuly described. Research has shown that the deficits in recent and remote memory, in the relative absence of other higher cortical dysfunction, are the hallmarks of the alcohol-related dementias. These memory deficits have specific characteristics that can be differentiated through neuropsychological testing from those seen in Alzheimer's disease (Moss et al 1986). Dementia associated with alcoholism is diagnosed when impairment involves other cognitive functions besides memory and is sufficient to interfere with social or occupational functioning.

CASE STUDY 7: DEPRESSION AND OTHER PSEUDODEMENTIAS

A 66-year-old, right-handed, retired administrative assistant was referred as a psychiatric inpatient for treatment of depression. He had a family history of affective disorder and had become clinically depressed after recent retirement and the death of his wife. On interview, he was psychomotorically slowed, was generally oriented (with effortful questioning), and appeared sad and despondent. His response to formal testing was generally cooperative but slowed. He frequently answered "I don't know" to questions and could not be motivated to respond. No particular asymmetries were noted, and constructional drawings were adequate although sparse. Attention and concentration were severely impaired. Verbal recall was adequate for recent news events, although the patient did poorly on formal memory tests. Abstract reasoning and topographical direction finding were reasonably intact. The history, clinical behavior, and cognitive test data strongly suggested depression rather than dementia, although the latter could not be ruled out. Personality testing suggested depression, not confusion. Vigorous treatment of depression was recommended.

Upon reevaluation a few weeks later, the patient's cognitive performance, psychomotor speed, and mood had improved measurably. A key diagnostic determinant in this man's history was that his cognitive impairment occurred abruptly *after* his losses (i.e., work and spouse). Had his cognitive impairment occurred first and in an insidious manner, as depression occurs frequently after a person recognizes progressive cognitive impairment, dementia and secondary, or reactive, depression would have been suspected more strongly.

Because virtually any medical illness can masquerade as dementia, a thorough history and complete medical evaluation are precursors to good diagnosis and treatment. In fact, treatment may reverse many treatable causes of dementia (i.e., psuedodementia). Neuropsychological testing is useful because it can help distinguish between cognitive impairment and emotional paralysis, as in depression, and can document quantitatively recovering or diminishing cognitive functioning over time. Memory complaints, for example, are very common among depressed elderly adults, and neuropsychological testing has been demonstrated to differentiate among patients with Alzheimer's disease, depression and normal control subjects on such factors as rates of forgetting (Hart et al 1987) and WAIS digit symbol performance (Hart et al 1987). Contrary to some anecdotal lore that demented patients do not appear depressed, patients in the early stages of dementia are frequently depressed to at least a mild degree, as shown by neuropsychological testing. In addition, many patients in chronic medical and/or psychiatric populations also have varying degrees of dementia (particularly milder forms) accompanying their chronic medical or psychiatric problems. Patients with medical problems may have, but are not limited to, cancer and vascular, lung, systemic, or neurological disease. The psychiatric groups that may have accompanying mild dementias are particularly comprised of chronic schizophrenias and affective and substance abuse disorders.

CASE STUDY 8: FOCAL LESIONS POSING AS DEMENTIA – THE ANGULAR GYRUS SYNDROME

A 52-year-old, right-handed, disabled auto mechanic with a high school education was referred as a medical outpatient because of memory problems and unpredictable behavior over the past 2 years. There was no definitive focal event in this man, who had a history of hypertension and occasional dizzy spells, but on close questioning his wife recalled one spell of dizziness after which his behavior seemed different. A long, premorbid history or intermittent alcohol abuse and antisocial behavior, such as spending and debauchery, complicated the history of behavioral change. There was no clear history of affective disorder. He had been "checked" by rural physicians but had not had a thorough evaluation for dementia.

A gregarious yet evasive character on interview, this patient's conversational speech suggested problems with language functions, comprehension being more affected than expression (fluency). For example, he engaged in overlearned, repetitive phrases such as, "You know what I mean . . . that's the way it goes," and otherwise had rather "empty," disjointed speech with approximately accurate phrasing (i.e., paraphasic). He had difficulty comprehending simple and complex commands and sometimes responded inappropriately. Reading, writing, calculation, and finger recognition were all impaired. Screening with the WAIS quickly revealed fairly good, although impaired, visuospatial and visuoconstructive skills on the block design subtest, but severely impaired language skills on the vocabulary subtest. Further testing of language and other cognitive functions supported the hypothesis of a posterior left cerebral hemisphere focal lesion, and a full medical workup with CT head scan was recommended to the referring resident physician. The CT scan revealed a lesion in the superior temporal gyrus of the left hemisphere, which was subsequently determined to be an old infarction (stroke) in Wernicke's area (and probably involved connecting pathways to the angular gyrus area), resulting in the syndrome of receptive/comprehension aphasia. As this man's condition had apparently not progressed significantly over the past 24 months, this was strongly suspected to be a case of a focal lesion seeming to be Alzheimer's disease.

Benson, Cummings, and Tsai (1982) reported a series of 75 difficult cases referred to the University of California-Los Angeles Neurobehavioral Service for further evaluation of dementia. Only 25% of these cases were subsequently found to involve Alzheimer's disease and 36% involved Multiinfarct dementia. Of the latter group half actually had what the authors called angular gyrus syndrome, a symptom complex resulting from lesions to the posterior left hemisphere. These symptoms, as in the case previously described, included fluent aphasia and difficulty reading, writing, calculating, recognizing fingers, and constructing. Although memory for verbal information was impaired, these patients typically could engage in complex social activities, retain the ability to know their way around, and so forth. This was true of the case with this patient, who continued to frustrate his wife with goal-directed yet sociopathic behavior. The neuropsychological evaluation aided in diagnosis and treatment planning, the wife's solicitation of family support, and follow-up at a local mental health center for assistance with management and family communication.

MALINGERING AND PSYCHOLOGICAL DYSFUNCTION

Patients occasionally feign or exaggerate cognitive problems, particularly those for whom there is a possibility of secondary gains, such as a decrease in personal responsibilities, escape from family conflict, or compensation for illness or incapacity. The neuropsychological evaluation is valuable in these cases because the standardized tests are good tools for detecting atypical patterns of performance, and malingering usually produces distinctly atypical patterns. For example, most patients are naive as to what variables constitute either a "normal" or abnormal performance, particularly in terms of what behavior and responses are typical of patients with Alzheimer's disease or multiinfarct dementia, the most common types of dementia. The Fuld profile on the WAIS is one example of empirical data that the typical patient would be unaware of and unable to replicate. This principle of interpretation is true of qualitative as well as quantitative aspects of the evaluation. That is, malingering behavior is often quite unusual in one or more ways.

In my experience, it is more likely to encounter patients who are exaggerating or distorting some real problems or deficits than faking illness altogether. The exaggeration is usually fairly obvious, in that they tend to endorse any and all symptoms inquired about, and symptom patterns and presentations do not follow known neuroanatomical pathways or functions. Deficits that are not consistent with neuroanatomical pathways and that are not reproducible on repeated trials are the hallmarks of malingering. Also, overly dramatic behavior is often evident, and test performance is disparately impaired compared with clinical behavior. For example, a patient will discuss his medical history in some detail, then declare on testing that he cannot recall his birthdate or address, recite the alphabet, or recall any details from a brief story, or he will feign some equally unlikely impairment that would be seen in only the most severely demented patient. Other nonverbal indications of manipulation, evasion, or deception, such as inconsistencies in information and/or behavior, are usually apparent.

Distinguishing malingering or obvious psychological dysfunction such as conversion hysteria from true brain dysfunction is usually less difficult than distinguishing subtle psychological factors affecting behavior, such as very mild depression, anxiety, or somatization disorders that may complicate and "overlay" real neurological dysfunction. Because these and other psychological symptoms such as irritability, fatigue, and emotional lability are characteristic of both dementia and psychological disorders and may occur in combination, the subtle distinctions are difficult. This is where a standardized group of tests in the hands of an experienced neuropsychologist is of unique value. As the growing body of literature in clinical neuropsychology expands and the number of practicing neuropsychologists increases, these evaluations and services are likely to become more available.

EMOTIONAL FACTORS

As described in the cases above, in the typical neuropsychological evaluation of dementia, much of the focus is on assessment of cognitive factors. Yet the importance of evaluating emotional variables should not be underestimated. Not only is this important when emotional variables are involved in the primary differential diagnosis, but the patient's and caregiver's reactions to the condition in question are always of critical importance, particularly in regard to treating and coping with the condition. Eventually, the neuropsychologist and other members of the interdisciplinary team typically devote nearly as much or more time working with the family or caregiver of the demented patient as with the patient.

Assessment of emotional factors can take two forms of evaluation. One is of the patient, the other is of the family system. In the former, the patient's objective mental status includes evaluation of emotionality. This may include formal testing of emotional variables and observations of emotionality during interviewing and cognitive testing. In early stages of dementia, the patient may be able to complete self-report inventories of feeling/personality, such as the Minnesota Multiphasic Personality Inventory (MMPI). More typically, the patient is too impaired to complete long questionnaires. Thus projective tests such as the Rorschach test may be useful. Although the Rorschach is not a good test of brain dysfunction per se, it can be helpful in eliciting and documenting empirically how a demented person is perceiving his environment. For example, the Rorschach helps determine whether a person has good contact with reality, how strongly he is affected by emotionality, and how effectively he is coping with it. Other projective tests may be used similarly, particularly when the variables in question are not sufficiently revealed by the other aspects of the evaluation. Such instruments may also help clarify the patient's subjective experience of emotionality in relation to his own personality or coping style, which can help individualize the treatment plan, particularly regarding individual and family psychotherapeutic interventions.

For example, the evaluation of a 57-year-old man with mild multiinfarct dementia and a right cerebral hemisphere stroke revealed that he had significant difficulty maintaining sustained attention and emotional control. He quickly changed topics of conversation, was impatient, and laughed or cried disinhibitedly with the slightest stimulation. His emotionality during the cognitive testing provided ample data that were used in later education of him and his wife in helping them cope with his problems. Personality testing with the patient and conjoint interviews with him and his wife helped elucidate emotional strengths, weaknesses, and communication patterns. For instance, personality testing revealed this patient's almost compulsive need to organize his environment and the painful affect he felt by being emotionally "out of control" even briefly, as well as his paternalistic relationship with his wife. This information was most helpful in constructing his individual treatment plan and the psychotherapeutic strategies with the couple.

Regarding the assessment of the family/caregiver system, inclusion of some form of assessment of the demented patient's support system is typically a necessary and important component of diagnosis and treatment. Although the patient's family may not significantly influence neuropathological factors, except perhaps regarding questions about the heritability of the disease, it certainly affects and is affected by the caregiver's reactions to the diagnosis and subsequent treatment plan. The diagnosis and treatment processes are effectually traumatic and stressful over time and include both the patient and the caregivers. As a result, models of diagnosis and treatment of the family system with a demented member flow naturally from the literatures of family psychotherapy and traumatic stress studies.

Figley (1988) proposed a model of treatment for families in traumatically stressful situations that drew on the work of others and combined aspects of general family systems theory, family psychotherapy and traumatic stress studies (Haly 1976; Minuchin 1976; Olson, Lavee, and McCubbin 1986). Most neuropsychologists or interdisciplinary team members who are trained psychotherapists use similar models, which involve systematic methods of evaluating and treating the broader family system. Such methods usually include evaluation of such factors as changing power structures in the family that accompany illness of a family member, the various dyadic (two-way) and triadic (three-way) relationships in the family, and communication systems within the family. Continuums of cohesion in the family and flexibility of roles, for example, are variables that can be evaluated, quantified, and employed in psychotherapeutic treatment during this time of stress. The degree of balance along either of the continuums can help predict how effectively a family will cope with such a stressful situation (Figley 1988).

This type of family evaluation does not imply that all families of demented patients are dysfunctional, pathological and in absolute need of psychotherapy. This merely represents a systematic way of evaluating and helping families of demented persons, regardless of their relative degree of "normalcy," because it is well known that a diagnosis of dementia is, at the very least, disturbing and potentially traumatic for even the most well-adjusted family.

Finally, a similar philosophy is applied to the evaluation of the family regarding potential referral to a support group. These groups can be quite informative and supportive for certain family members and caregivers. Thus attention to evaluation of the individual family member's suitability for specific referrals (e.g., traditional support group versus psychotherapy group) can be beneficial. The success or degree of helpfulness obtained by the member may well be related to the appropriateness, timeliness, and individual attention given to the referral process. This issue emphasizes the neuropsychologist's and team's effort not to overlook or focus too specifically on either the patient or the caregivers to the exclusion of the other in the diagnostic and treatment planning process.

SUMMARY

The neuropsychological evaluation of dementia is typically a comprehensive endeavor involving various methods, instrumentation, and focuses. Clearly the diagnostic aspects of the evaluation focus more on cognitive factors, by their historical and natural role, whereas the treatment aspects include more emphasis on emotional, interpersonal, and family factors. This requires a combination of clinical skill, relatively precise measurement, and psychotherapeutic acumen. Any given referral question may require one or more aspects of the evaluation to be emphasized. The foregoing description and case examples have highlighted both the traditional and developing issues to be addressed by the typical neuropsychological evaluation of dementia.

BIBLIOGRAPHY

American Psychiatric Association: Diagnostic and statistical manual of mental disorders, ed 3, Washington, DC, 1987, The Association.

Benson DF, Cummings JL, and Tsai SY: Angular gyrus syndrome simulating Alzheimer's disease, Arch Neurol 39:616-620, 1982.

Benton AL et al: Contributions to neuropsychological assessment, New York, 1983, Oxford University Press.

Figley CR: A five-phase treatment of post-traumatic stress disorder in families, J Traumatic Stress 1:127-141, 1988.

Fillenbaum GG et al: Comparison of two screening tests in Alzheimer's disease, Arch Neurol 44:924-927, 1987.

Fisk AA et al: Alzheimer's disease: a five article symposium, Postgrad Med 73:204-256, 1983.

Friedland RP et al: NIH conference—Alzheimer's disease: clinical and biological heterogeneity, Ann Inter Med 109(4):298-311, 1980.

Fuld PA: Psychometric differentiation of the dementias: an overview. In Reisberg B, editor: Alzheimer's disease. New York, 1983, MacMillan, Inc.

Fuld PA et al: Intrusions as a sign of Alzheimer's dementia: chemical and pathological verification, Ann Neurol 11:155-159, 1982.

Golden CJ: A standardized version of Luria's neuropsychological tests. In Filskov S and Boll TJ, editors: Handbook of clinical neuropsychology, New York, 1981, Wiley-Interscience.

Hachinski VC et al: Cerebral blood flow in dementia, Arch Neurol 32:632-637, 1975.

Haley J: Problem-solving therapy, San Francisco, 1976, Jossey-Bass, Inc, Publishers.

Hart RP et al: Digit symbol performance in mild dementia and depression, J Consult Clin Psychol 55:236-238, 1987a.

Hart RP et al: Rate of forgetting in dementia and depression, J Consult Clin Psychol 55:101-105, 1987b.

Huber SJ et al: Cortical versus subcortical dementia: neuropsychological differences, Arch Neurol 43:392-394, 1986.

Katzman RD: Alzheimer's disease, N Engl J Med 314:964-973, 1986.

Katzman R et al: Validation of a short orientation-memory-concentration test of cognitive impairment, Am J Psychiatry 140:734-739, 1983.

Lesher EL and Whelihan WM: Reliability of mental status instruments administered to nursing home residents, J Consult Clin Psychol 54:726-727, 1987.

Luria AR: Higher cortical functions in man, New York, 1966, Basic Books.

Mayeaux et al: Is "subcortical dementia" a recognizable clinical entity? Ann Neurol 14:278-283, 1983.

Minuchin S: Families and family therapy, Cambridge, Mass, 1974, Harvard University Press.

Moss MB et al: Differential patterns of memory loss among patients with Alzheimer's disease, Huntington's disease, and alcoholic Korsakoff's syndrome, Arch Neurol 43:239-246, 1986.

Navia BA Jordan BD, and Price RW: The AIDS dementia complex: I. Clinical features, Ann Neurol 19, 517-524, 1986.

Navia BA and Price RW: The acquired immunodeficiency syndrome dementia complex as the presenting sole manifestation of human immunodeficiency virus infection, Arch Neurol 44:65, 1987.

Olson DH, Lavee Y, and McCubbin HI: Types of families and family response to stress across the family life cycle. In Aldous J and Klein DM, editors: Social stress and family development, New York, 1986, Gilford Press.

Reitan RM and Wolfson D: The Halstead-Reitan neuropsychological test battery: theory and clinical interpretation, Tucson, 1985, Neuropsychological Press.

Rosen WG et al: Pathological verification of ischemic score in differentiation of dementias, Ann Neurol 7:486-488, 1980.

Sloan P: Clinical neuropsychology in evaluating and treating brain dysfunction, South Med J 77:4-6, 1984.

Suggested readings

REVIEW ARTICLES

Abernethy DR: Development of memory-enhancing agents in the treatment of Alzheimer's disease, J Am Geriatr Soc 35:957, 1987.

Amaducci L and Lippi A: Risk factors and genetic background for Alzheimer's disease, Acta Neurol Scand (Suppl) 116:13-18, 1988.

Berg L: Mild senile dementia of the Alzheimer's type: diagnostic criteria and natural history, Mt Sinai J Med (NY) 55(1):87-96, 1988.

Billig N: Alzheimer's disease. A psychiatrist's perspective, Nurs Clin North Am 23(1):125-133, 1988.

Blackburn IM and Tyrer GM: The value of Luria's neuropsychological investigation for the assessment of cognitive dysfunction in Alzheimer-type dementia. Part III, Br J Clin Psychol 24:171-179, 1985.

Boller F, Lopez OL, and Moossy J: Diagnosis of dementia: clinicopathologic correlations, Neurology 39(1):76-79, 1989.

Brayne C and Calloway P: Normal ageing, impaired cognitive function, and senile dementia of the Alzheimer's type: a continuum? Lancet 1(8597):1265-1267, 1988.

Burns EM and Buckwalter KC: Pathophysiology and etiology of Alzheimer's disease, Nurs Clin North Am 23(1):11-29, 1988.

Carrell RW: Alzheimer's disease. Enter a protease inhibitor, Nature 331(6156):478-479, 1988.

Castano EM and Frangione B: Human amyloidosis, Alzheimer disease and related disorders, Lab Invest 58(2):122-132, 1988.

Claggett MS: Nutritional factors relevant to Alzheimer's disease, J Am Diet Assoc 89(3):392-396, 1989.

Clarfield AM: The reversible dementias: do they reverse? Ann Intern Med 109(6):476-486, 1988.

Constantinidis J, Bouras C, and Vallet PG: Neuropeptides in Alzheimer's and Parkinson's disease, Mt Sinai J Med (NY) 55(1):102-115, 1988.

Coyle JT, Price DL, and DeLong MR: Alzheimer's disease: a disorder of cortical cholinergic innervation, Science 219(4589):1184-1190, 1983.

Crook T et al, editors: Treatment development strategies for Alzheimer's disease, Madison, Conn, 1986, Mark Pawley.

Cross PS, Gurland BJ, and Mann AH: Long-term institutional care of demented elderly people in New York City and London, Bull NY Acad Med 59(3):267-275, 1983.

Cummings JL: The dementias of Parkinson's disease: prevalence, characteristics, neurobiology, and comparison with dementia of the Alzheimer type, Eur Neurol 28 (suppl 1):15-23, 1988.

Cummings JL et al: Aphasia in dementia of the Alzheimer type, Neurology 35(3):394-397, 1985.

Cutler NR et al: NIH Conference. Alzheimer's disease and Down's syndrome: new insights, Ann Intern Med 103(4):566-578, 1985.

Davidson M et al: Endocrine changes in Alzheimer' disease, Neurol Clin 6(1):149-157, 1988.

Davies P: Neurochemical studies: an update on Alzheimer's disease, J Clin Psychiatry 49 suppl:23-28, 1988.

Davis KL and Mohs RC: Cholinergic drugs in Alzheimer's disease, N Engl J Med 315(20):1286-1287, 1986.

Deary IJ and Whalley LJ: Recent research on the causes of Alzheimer's disease, Br Med J 297(6652):807-810, 1988.

Drayer BP: Imaging of the aging brain. II. Pathologic conditions, Radiology 166(3):797-806, 1988.

Farooqui AA, Liss L, and Horrocks LA: Neurochemical aspects of Alzheimer's disease: involvement of membrane phospholipids, Metab Brain Dis 3(1):19-35, 1988.

Filley CM: Diagnosis of Alzheimer's disease, Colo Med 85(3):48-49, 1988.

Fisk AA: Management of Alzheimer's disease, Postgrad Med 73(4):237-241, 1983.

Friedland RP et al: NIH conference. Alzheimer disease: clinical and biological heterogeneity, Ann Intern Med 109(4):298-311, 1988.

Gado MH and Press GA: Computed tomography in the diagnosis of dementia, Geriatric Medicine Today 5(7):47-73, 1986.

Gauthier S: Practical guidelines for the antemortem diagnosis of senile dementia of the Alzheimer type, Prog Neuropsychopharmacol Biol Psychiatry 9(5-6):491-495, 1985.

Glenner GG: Alzheimer's disease: its proteins and genes, Cell 52(3):307-308, 1988.

Gottfries CG: Alzheimer's disease and senile dementia: biochemical characteristics and aspects of treatment, Psychopharmacology 86:245-252, 1985.

Gottfries CG: Dementia: classification and aspects of treatment, Psychopharmacol Ser 5:187-195, 1988.

Gottlieb GL, McAllister TW and Gur RC: Depot neuroleptics in the treatment of behavioral disorders in patients with Alzheimer's disease, J Am Geriatr Soc 36:619-621, 1988.

Gray-Vickrey P: Evaluating Alzheimer's patients: the importance of being thorough, Nursing '88 18(12):34-42, 1988.

Green JA: Alzheimer's disease: practical aspects, Intern Med 8(6):181-193, 1987.

Greenwald BS, Mohs RC, and Davis KL: Neurotransmitter deficits in Alzheimer's disease: criteria for significance, J Am Geriatr Soc 31(5):310-316, 1983.

Hall GR: Care of the patient with Alzheimer's disease living at home, Nurs Clin North Am 23(1):31-46, 1988.

Hamill RW et al: Neurodegenerative disorders and aging. Alzheimer's disease and Parkinson's disease — common ground, Ann NY Acad Sci 515:411-420, 1988.

Hardy J: Molecular biology and Alzheimer's disease: more questions than answers [news], Trends Neurosci 11(7):293-294, 1988.

Hardy JA and Davies DC: Alzheimer's disease, Br J Hosp Med 39(5):372-373, 376-377, 1988.

Haycox JA: Management of a demented patient, Bull NY Acad Med 59(3):262-266, 1983.

Henderson AS: The risk factors for Alzheimer's disease: a review and a hypothesis, Acta Psychiatr Scand 78(3):257-275, 1988.

Henderson VW and Finch CE: The neurobiology of Alzheimer's disease, J Neurosurg 70(3):335-353, 1989.

Heston LL: Down's syndrome and Alzheimer's dementia: defining and association, Psychiatr Dev 2(4):287-294, 1984.

Homer AC et al: Diagnosing dementia: do we get it right? BMJ 297(6653):894-896, 1988.

Kaszniak AW: Cognition in Alzheimer's disease: theoretic models and clinical implications, Neurobiol Aging 9(1):92-94, 1988.

Katzman R: Alzheimer's disease, N Engl J Med 314(15):964-973, 1986.

Katzman R: Alzheimer's disease as an age-dependent disorder, Ciba Found Symp 134:69-85, 1988.

Kim KY and Hershey LA: Diagnosis and treatment of depression in the elderly, Int J Psychiatry Med 18(3):211-221, 1988.

Koranyi EK: The cortical dementias, Can J Psychiatry 33(9):838-845, 1988.

Larson EB, Lo B, and Williams ME: Evaluation and care of elderly patients with dementia, J Gen Intern Med 1(Mar/Apr):116-129, 1986.

Lo B and Dornbrand L: Guiding the hand that feeds: Caring for the demented elderly, N Engl J Med 311(6):402-404, 1984.

Lott IT: Down's syndrome, aging, and Alzheimer's disease: a clinical review, Ann NY Acad Sci 396:15-27, 1982.

Mann DM: Alzheimer's disease and Down's syndrome, Histopathology 13(2):125-137, 1988.

Martin RA and Guthrie R: Office evaluation of dementia. How to arrive at a clear diagnosis and choose appropriate therapy, Postgrad Med 84(3):176-180, 183-187, 1988.

McClelland L: Alzheimer's disease: a savage master, Geriatr Nur Home Care 8(11-12):22-24, 1988.

McKhann G et al: Clinical diagnosis of Alzheimer's disease: report of the NINCDS-ADRDA Work Group, Neurology 34:939-944, 1984.

McLachlan DR and Lewis PN: Alzheimer's disease: errors in gene expression, Can J Neurol Sci 12(1):1-5, 1985.

Merriam AE et al: The psychiatric symptoms of Alzheimer's disease, J Am Geriatr Soc 36(1):7-12, 1988.

Merskey H et al: Correlative studies in Alzheimer's disease, Prog Neuropsychopharmacol Biol Psychiatry 9(5-6):509-514, 1985.

Morris JC and Fulling K: Early Alzheimer's disease. Diagnostic considerations, Arch Neurol 45(3):345-349, 1988.

Morris RG and Baddeley AD: Primary and working memory functioning in Alzheimer-type dementia, J Clin Exp Neuropsychol 10(2):279-296, 1988.

Moss RJ, Mastri AR, and Schut LJ: The coexistence and differentiation of late onset Huntington's disease and Alzheimer's disease. A case report and review of the literature, J Am Geriatr Soc 36(3):237-241, 1988.

Overman W Jr and Stoudemire A: Guidelines for legal and financial counseling of Alzheimer's disease patients and their families, Am J Psychiatry 145(12):1495-1500, 1988.

Parker JC Jr and Philpot J: Postmortem evaluation of Alzheimer's disease, South Med J 78(12):1411-1413, 1985.

Price DL et al: Neurobiological studies of transmitter systems in aging and in Alzheimer-type dementia, Ann NY Acad Sci 457:35-51, 1985.

Procter AW et al: Topographical distribution of neurochemical changes in Alzheimer's disease, J Neurol Sci 84(2-3):125-140, 1988.

Rapoport SI: Brain evolution and Alzheimer's disease, Rev Neurol (Paris) 144(2):79-90, 1988.

Reifler BV and Larson EB: Alzheimer's disease and long-term care: the assessment of the patient, J Geriatr Psychiatry 18(1):9-35, 1985.

Riege WH and Metter EJ: Cognitive and brain imaging measures of Alzheimer's disease, Neurobiol Aging 9(1):69-86, 1985.

Rocca WA and Amaducci L: The familial aggregation of Alzheimer's disease: an epidemiological review, Psychiatr Dev 6(1):23-36, 1988.

Rosen WG, Mohs RC, and Davis KL: A new rating scale for Alzheimer's disease, Am J Psychiatry 141(11):1356-1364, 1984.

Rousseau P: Binswanger's disease: a cause of dementia in the elderly, South Med J 81(10):1329-1330, 1988.

Rubin EH, Zorumski CF, and Burke WJ: Overlapping symptoms of geriatric depression and Alzheimer-type dementia, Hosp Community Psychiatry 39(10):1074-1079, 1988.

Scarone S et al: Neurofunctional assessment of early phases of Alzheimer's disease: a preliminary note on hemispheric EEG characteristics during cognitive tasks, Hum Neurobiol 6(4):289-293, 1988.

Senile dementia of Alzheimer's type—normal ageing or disease? (editorial), Lancet 1(8636):476-477, 1989.

Singh S, Mulley GP, and Losowsky MS: Why are Alzheimer patients thin? Age Ageing 17:21-28, 1988.

Skullerud K: Variations in the size of the human brain. Influence of age, sex, body length, body mass index, alcoholism, Alzheimer changes, and cerebral atherosclerosis, Acta Neurol Scand (Suppl) 102:1-94, 1985.

Small GW and Greenberg DA: Biologic markers, genetics, and Alzheimer's disease, Arch Gen Psychiatry 45(10):945-947, 1988.

Smith G: Animal models of Alzheimer's disease: experimental cholinergic denervation, Brain Res 472(2):103-118, 1988.

Spinnler H and Della Sala S: The role of clinical neuropsychology in the neurological diagnosis of Alzheimer's disease, J Neurol 235(5):258-271, 1988.

Thal LJ: Dementia update: diagnosis and neuropsychiatric aspects, J Clin Psychiatry 49 (supp):5-7, 1988.

Thienhaus OJ et al: Biologic markers in Alzheimer's disease, J Am Geriatr Soc 33(10):715-726, 1985.

Toledano-Gasca A: Hypotheses concerning the aetiology of Alzheimer's disease, Pharmacopsychiatry 21 (suppl) 1:17-25, 1988.

Uhlmann RF et al: Impact of mild to moderate hearing loss on mental status testing. Comparability of standard and written Mini-Mental State Examinations, J Am Geriatr Soc 37(3):223-228, 1989.

Volicer L et al: Hospice approach to the treatment of patients with advanced dementia of the Alzheimer type, JAMA 256:2210-2213, 1986.

Wilcock GK: Alzheimer's disease—current issues, QJ Med 66(250):117-124, 1988.

Winograd CH and Jarvik LF: Physician management of the demented patient, J Am Geriatr Soc 34:295-308, 1986.

Wisniewski HM and Wrzolek M: Pathogenesis of amyloid formation in Alzheimer's disease, Down's syndrome and scrapie, Ciba Found Symp 135:224-238, 1988.

Zimmer R and Lauter H: Diagnosis, differential diagnosis and nosologic classification of the dementia syndrome, Pharmacopsychiatry 21 (suppl) 1:1-7, 1988.

ORIGINAL ARTICLES

Agbayewa MO: Earlier psychiatric morbidity in patients with Alzheimer's disease, J Am Geriatr Soc 34:561-564, 1986.

Aharon-Peretz J, Cummings JL, and Hill MA: Vascular dementia and dementia of the Alzheimer type, Arch Neurol 45(7):719-721, 1988.

Altman J: A nose for Alzheimer's disease? [news] Nature 337(6209):688, 1989.

Ball MJ et al: Neuropathological definition of Alzheimer disease: multivariate analyses in the morphometric distinction between Alzheimer dementia and normal aging, Alzheimer Dis Assoc Disord 2(1):29-37, 1988.

Bayles KA et al: Differentiating Alzheimer's patients from the normal elderly and stroke patients with aphasia, J Speech Hear Disord 54(1):74-87, 1989.

Beach TG: The history of Alzheimer's disease: three debates, J Hist Med Allied Sci 42:327-349, 1987.

Beal MF et al: Widespread reduction of somatostatin-like immunoreactivity in the cerebral cortex in Alzheimer's disease, Ann Neurol 20:489-495, 1986.

Beck C and Heacock P: Nursing interventions for patients with Alzheimer's disease, Nurs Clin North Am 23(1):95-124, 1988.

Becker JT et al: Neuropsychological function in Alzheimer's disease. Pattern of impairment and rates of progression, Arch Neurol 45(3):263-268, 1988.

Beller SA et al: Long-term outpatient treatment of senile dementia with oral physostigmine, J Clin Psychiatry 49(10):400-404, 1988.

Berg L et al: Mild senile dementia of the Alzheimer type: II. Longitudinal assessment, Ann Neurol 23(5):477-484, 1988.

Berrettini WH et al: Galanin immunoreactivity in human CSF: studies in eating disorders and Alzheimer's disease, Neuropsychobiology 19(2):64-68, 1988.

Bird TD et al: Phenotypic heterogeneity in familial Alzheimer's disease: a study of 24 kindreds, Ann Neurol 25(1):12-25, 1989,

Blackwood DHR and Christie JE: The efffects of physostigmine on memory and auditory P300 in Alzheimer-type dementia, Biol Psychiatry 21:557-560, 1986.

Blass JP et al: Thiamine and Alzheimer's disease. A pilot study, Arch Neurol 45(8):833-835, 1988.

Bliwise DL et al: REM latency in Alzheimer's disease, Biol Psychiatry 25(3):320-328, 1989.

Bonte FJ et al: The effect of acetazolamide on regional cerebral blood flow in patients with Alzheimer's disease or stroke as measured by single-photon emission computed tomography, Invest Radiol 24(2):99-103, 1989.

Borson S et al: Impaired sympathetic nervous system response to cognitive effort in early Alzheimer's disease, J Gerontol 44(1):M8-12, 1989.

Botwinick J Storandt M, and Berg L: A longitudinal, behavioral study of senile dementia of the Alzheimer type, Arch Neurol 43:1124-1127, 1986.

Brandt J et al: Semantic activation and implicit memory in Alzheimer disease, Alzheimer Dis Assoc Disord 2(2):112-119, 1988.

Broks P et al: Modelling dementia: effects of scopolamine on memory and attention, Neuropsychologia 26(5):685-700, 1988.

Buhl L and Bojsen-Mller M: Frequency of Alzheimer's disease in a postmortem study of psychiatric patients, Dan Med Bull 35(3):288-290, 1988.

Cacabelos R et al: Influence of somatostatin and growth hormone-releasing factor on behavior. Clinical and therapeutic implications in neuropsychiatric disorders, Horm Res 29(2-3):129-312, 1988.

Cadet JL: A unifying theory of movement and madness: involvement of free radicals in disorders of the isodendritic core of the brainstem, Med Hypotheses 27(1):59-63, 1988.

Chan-Palay V: Galanin hyperinnervates surviving neurons of the human basal nucleus of Meynert in dementias of Alzheimer's and Parkinson's disease: a hypothesis for the role of galanin in accentuating cholinergic dysfunction in dementia, J Comp Neurol 273(4):543-557, 1988.

Chandler JD and Gerndt J: Cognitive screening tests for organic mental disorders in psychiatric inpatients. A hopeless task? J Nerv Ment Dis 176(11):675-681, 1988.

Christie JE et al: Magnetic resonance imaging in pre-senile dementia of the Alzheimer-type, multi-infarct dementia and Korsakoff's syndrome, Psychol Med 18(2):319-329, 1988.

Cleary TA et al: A reduced stimulation unit: effects on patients with Alzheimer's disease and related disorders, Gerontologist 28(4):511-514, 1988.

Colerick EJ and George LK: Predictors of institutionalization among caregivers of patients with Alzheimer's disease, J Am Geriatr Soc 34:493-498, 1986.

Cortes R, Probst A, and Palacios JM: Decreased densities of dopamine D1 receptors in the putamen and hippocampus in senile dementia of the Alzheimer type, Brain Res 475(1):164-167, 1988.

Cowburn JD and Blair JA: Aluminium chelator (transferrin) reverses biochemical deficiency in Alzheimer brain preparations, Lancet 1(8629):99, 1989 (letter).

Cutler NR: Cognitive and brain imaging measures of Alzheimer's disease, Neurobiol Aging 9(1):90-92, 1988.

David F, Clerget F, and Lucote G: Familial Alzheimer's disease (FAD): co-segregation between alleles at the D21S11 DNA marker and the FAD gene in a particular pedigree, J Neurol 235(8):485-486, 1988.

Davies L et al: A4 amyloid protein deposition and the diagnosis of Alzheimer's disease: prevalence in aged brains determined by immunocytochemistry compared with conventional neuropathologic techniques, Neurology 38(11):1688-1693, 1988.

Davous P and Lamour Y: Bethanechol decreases reaction time in senile dementia of the Alzheimer type, J Neurol Neurosurg Psychiatry 48:1297-1299, 1985.

Deimling GT and Bass DM: Symptoms of mental impairment among elderly adults and their effects on family caregivers, J Ger 41:(6):778-784, 1986.

De Leo D, Schifano F, and Magni G: Results of dexamethasone suppression test in early Alzheimer dementia, Eur Arch Psychiatry Neurol Sci 238(1):19-21, 1988.

De Leon MJ et al: Positron emission tomography with the deoxyglucose technique and the diagnosis of Alzheimer's disease, Neurobiol Aging 9(1):88-90, 1988.

Degrell I and Niklasson F: Purine metabolites in the CSF in presenile and senile dementia of Alzheimer type, and in multi-infarct dementia, Arch Gerontol Geriatr 7(2):173-178, 1988.

Dick MB, Kean ML, and Sands D: Memory for action events in Alzheimer-type dementia: further evidence of an encoding failure, Brain Cogn 9(1):71-87, 1989.

Dick MB, Kean ML, and Sands D: Memory for internally generated words in Alzheimer-type dementia: breakdown in encoding and semantic memory, Brain Cogn 9(1):88-108, 1989.

Doebler JA et al: Neuronal RNA in Pick's and Alzheimer's diseases. Comparison of disease-susceptible and disease-resistant cortical areas, Arch Neurol 46(2):134-137, 1989.

Drevets WC and Rubin EH: Psychotic symptoms and the longitudinal course of senile dementia of the Alzheimer type, Biol Psychiatry 25(1):39-48, 1989.

Edlin GJ: The senile dementias: a new model, Med Hypotheses 27(1):29-31, 1989.

Englund E, Brun A, and Alling C: White matter changes in dementia of Alzheimer's type. Biochemical and neuropathological correlates. Part 6, Brain 111:1425-1439, 1988.

Erde EL, Nadal EC, and Scholl TO: On truth telling and the diagnosis of Alzheimer's disease, J Fam Pract 26(4):401-406, 1988.

Erkinjuntti T et al: EEG in the differential diagnosis between Alzheimer's disease and vascular dementia, Acta Neurol Scand 77(1):36-43, 1988.

Erkinjuntti T, Sulkava R, and Tilvis R: Is determination of plasma lipids useful in the differentiation of multi-infarct dementia from Alzheimer's disease? Compr Gerontol [A] 2(1):1-6, 1988.

Fabiszewski KJ: Caring for the Alzheimer's patient, Gerodontology 6(2):53-58, 1987.

Farber JF, Schmitt FA, and Logue PE: Predicting intellectual level from the Mini-Mental State Examination, J Am Geriatr Soc 36(6):509-510, 1988.

Filley CM, Kelly J, and Heaton RK: Neuropsychologic features of early- and late-onset Alzheimer's disease, Arch Neurol 43:574-576, 1986.

Filley CM et al: A comparison of dementia in Alzheimer's disease and multiple sclerosis, Arch Neurol 46(2):157-161, 1989.

Fisher P, Gatterer G, and Danielczyk W: Semantic memory in DAT, MID and parkinsonism, Funct Neurol 3(3):301-307, 1988.

Fischer P et al: Nonspecificity of semantic impairment in dementia of Alzheimer's type, Arch Neurol 45(12):1341-1343, 1988.

Fitch N, Becker R, and Heller A: The inheritance of Alzheimer's disease: a new interpretation, Ann Neurol 23(1):14-19, 1988.

Flaten TP and Odegard M: Tea, aluminium and Alzheimer's disease, Food Chem Toxicol 26(11-12):959-960, 1988 (letter).

Foley P et al: Evidence for the presence of antibodies to cholinergic neurons in the serum of patients with Alzheimer's disease, J Neurol 235(8):466-471, 1988.

Franceschi M et al: Neuroendocrinological function in Alzheimer's disease, Neuroendocrinology 48(4):367-370, 1988.

Freed DM and Kandel E: Long-term occupational exposure and the diagnosis of dementia, Neurotoxicology 9(3):391-400, 1988.

Freedman M and Oscar-Berman M: Selective delayed response deficits in Parkinson's and Alzheimer's disease, Arch Neurol 43:886-890, 1986.

Freund G and Ballinger WE Jr: Loss of cholinergic muscarinic receptors in the frontal cortex of alcohol abusers, Alcoholism (NY) 12(5):630-638, 1988.

Friedland RP, et al: Measurement of disease progression in Alzheimer's disease, Neurobiol Aging 9(1):95-97, 1988.

Friedland RP et al: Motor vehicle crashes in dementia of the Alzheimer type, Ann Neurol 24(6):782-786, 1988.

Gagnon M et al: Predictors of non-bedridden survival in dementia, Eur Neurol 28(5):270-274, 1988.

Gambert SR: Dementia secondary to metabolic and nutritional abnormalities, Clin Geriatr Med 4(4):831-839, 1988.

Gauthier S et al: Transmitter-replacement therapy in Alzheimer's disease using intracerebroventricular infusions of receptor agonists, Can J Neurol Sci 13:394-402, 1986.

Gemmell HG et al: A comparison of Tc-99m HM-PAO and I-123 IMP cerebral SPECT images in Alzheimer's disease and multi-infarct dementia, Eur J Nucl Med 14(9-10):463-466, 1988.

Giaccone G et al: Down patients: extracellular preamyloid deposits precede neuritic degeneration and senile plaques, Neurosci Lett 97(1-2):232-238, 1989.

Goate AM et al: Predisposing locus for Alzheimer's disease on chromosome 21, Lancet 1(8634):352-355, 1989.

Goodman CC and Pynoos J: Telephone networks connect caregiving families of Alzheimer's victims, Gerontologist 28(5):602-605, 1988.

Gottlieb GL, Gur RE, and Gur RC: Reliability of psychiatric scales in patients with dementia of the Alzheimer type, Am J Psychiatry 145(7):857-860, 1988.

Grady CL et al: Divided attention, as measured by dichotic speech performance, in dementia of the Alzheimer type, Arch Neurol 46(3):317-320, 1989.

Grady CL, et al: Longitudinal study of the early neuropsychological and cerebral metabolic changes in dementia of the Alzheimer type, J Clin Exp Neuropsychol 10(5):576-596, 1988.

Greenamyre JT et al: Glutamate transmission and toxicity in Alzheimer's disease, Prog Neuropsychopharmacol Biol Psychiatry 12(4):421-430, 1988.

Guralnik JM and Branch LG: Direct assessment of ADL in Alzheimer's disease, J Am Geriatr Soc 37(2):196-197, 1989 (letter).

Hammerstrom DC and Zimmer B: The role of lumbar puncture in the evaluation of dementia: the University of Pittsburgh study, J Am Geriatr Soc 33(6):397-400, 1985.

Haxby JV et al: Neocortical metabolic abnormalities precede nonmemory cognitive defects in early Alzheimer's-type dementia, Arch Neurol 43:882-885, 1986.

Hefti F and Weiner WJ: Nerve growth factor and Alzheimer's disease, Ann Neurol 20:275-281, 1986.

Heindel WC et al: Neuropsychological evidence for multiple implicit memory systems: a comparison of Alzheimer's, Huntington's, and Parkinson's disease patients, J Neurosci 9(2):582-587, 1989.

Hepburn KW and Gates BA: Family caregivers for non-Alzheimer's dementia patients, Clin Geriatr Med 4(4):925-940, 1988.

Heyman A et al: Alzheimer's disease: a study of epidemiological aspects, Ann Neurol 15:335-341, 1984.

Hoch CC et al: Clinical significance of sleep-disordered breathing in Alzheimer's disease. Preliminary data, J Am Geriatr Soc 37(2):138-144, 1989.

Howell M: Caretakers' views on responsibilities for the care of the demented elderly, J Am Geriatr Soc 32(9):657-660, 1984.

Huber SJ et al: Cortical vs subcortical dementia, Arch Neurol 43:392-394, 1986.

Huff FJ et al: Risk of dementia in relatives of patients with Alzheimer's disease, Neurology 38(5):786-790, 1988.

Ikeda S, Allsop D, and Glenner GG: Morphology and distribution of plaque and related deposits in the brains of Alzheimer's disease and control cases. An immunohistochemical study using amyloid beta-protein antibody, Lab Invest 60(1):113-122, 1989.

Janota I and Mountjoy CQ: Asymmetry of pathology in Alzheimer's disease, J Neurol Neurosurg Psychiatry 51(7):1011-1012, 1988 (letter).

Joachim CL, Morris JH, and Selkoe DJ: Clinically diagnosed Alzheimer's disease: autopsy results in 150 cases, Ann Neurol 24(1):50-56, 1988.

Johnson CC: Occurrence of Alzheimer disease in Michigan: an epidemiologic review of rates and risk factors, Henry Ford Hosp Med J 36(2):117-120, 1988.

Kaszniak AW: Cognition in Alzheimer's disease: theoretic models and clinical implications, Neurobiol Aging 9(1):92-94, 1988.

Katz SI et al: The effects of a day respite program on caregiver health, VA Practitioner 4(11):49-59, 1987.

Katzman R et al: Comparison of rate of annual change of mental status score in four independent studies of patients with Alzheimer's disease, Ann Neurol 24(3):384-389, 1988.

Kempler D, Van Lancker D, and Read S: Proverb and idiom comprehension in Alzheimer disease, Alzheimer Dis Assoc Disord 2(1):38-49, 1988.

Kesner RP: Reevaluation of the contribution of the basal forebrain cholinergic system to memory, Neurobiol Aging 9(5-6):609-616, 1988.

Kiecolt-Glaser JK, Dyer CS, and Shuttleworth EC: Upsetting social interactions and distress among Alzheimer's disease family care-givers: a replication and extension, Am J Community Psychol 16(6):825-837, 1988.

Kingsley BS, Gaskin F, and Fu SM: Human antibodies to neurofibrillary tangles and astrocytes in Alzheimer's disease, J Neuroimmunol 19(1-2):89-99, 1988.

Klein LE et al: Diagnosing dementia. Univariate and multivariate analyses of the mental status examination, J Am Geriatr Soc 33:483-488, 1985.

Knight RG and Moroney BM: An investigation of the validity of the Kendrick Battery for the detection of dementia in the elderly, International J Clin Neuropsych 7(3):147-151, 1984.

Knopman DS and Ryberg S: A verbal memory test with high predictive accuracy for dementia of the Alzheimer type, Arch Neurol 46(2):141-145, 1989.

Kosaka K, Tsuchiya K, and Yoshimura M: Lewy body disease with and without dementia: a clinicopathological study of 35 cases, Clin Neuropathol 7(6):299-305, 1988.

Kumar M, Cohen D, and Eisdorfer C: Serum IgG brain reactive antibodies in Alzheimer disease and Down syndrome, Alzheimer Dis Assoc Disord 2(1):50-55, 1988.

Kurlan R and Como P: Drug-induced alzheimerism, Arch Neurol 45(3):356-357, 1988.

Landfield PW: Hippocampal neurobiological mechanisms of age-related memory dysfunction, Neurobiol Aging 9(5-6):571-579, 1988.

Larson EB et al: Diagnostic evaluation of 200 elderly outpatients with suspected dementia, J Gerontol 40(5):536-543, 1985.

Lecso PA: Murder-suicide in Alzheimer's disease, J Am Geriatr Soc 37(2):167-168, 1989.

Leonardi A et al: Functional study of T lymphocyte responsiveness in patients with dementia of the Alzheimer type, J Neuroimmunol 22(1):19-22, 1989.

Lewis AJ et al: Pathologic diagnosis of Alzheimer's disease, Neurology 38(10):1660, 1988 (letter).

Loewenstein DA et al: Predominant left hemisphere metabolic dysfunction in dementia, Arch Neurol 46(2):146-152, 1989.

Loring DW and Largen JW: Neuropsychological patterns of presenile and senile dementia of the Alzheimer type, Neuropsychologia 23(3):351-357, 1985.

Maletta GJ: Management of behavior problems in elderly patients with Alzheimer's disease and other dementias, Clin Geriatr Med 4(4):719-747, 1988.

Marta M et al: New analogs of physostigmine: alternative drugs for Alzheimer's disease? Life Sci 43(23):1921-1928, 1988.

Martyn CN et al: Geographical relation between Alzheimer's disease and aluminum in drinking water, Lancet 1(8629):59-62, 1989.

Matsuyama SS and Bohman R: Variation in DNA content of mononuclear cells of patients with dementia of the Alzheimer type, Alzheimer Dis Assoc Disord 2(2):120-122, 1988.

Matsuyama SS and Fu TK: Sister chromatid exchanges and dementia of the Alzheimer type, Neurobiol Aging 9(4):405-408, 1988.

McGrowder-Lin R and Bhatt A: A Wanderer's Lounge Program for nursing home residents with Alzheimer's disease, Gerontologist 28(5):607-609, 1988.

McGeer PL et al: Reactive microglia are positive for HLA-DR in the substantia nigra of Parkinson's and Alzheimer's disease brains, Neurology 38(8):1285-1291, 1988.

McGeer PL et al: Occurrence of HLA-DR reactive microglia in Alzheimer's disease, Ann N Y Acad Sci 540:319-323, 1988.

Merriam AE et al: The psychiatric symptoms of Alzheimer's disease, J Am Geriatr Soc 36:7-12, 1988.

Mesulam MM and Geula C: Acetylcholinesterase-rich pyramidal neurons in the human neocortex and hippocampus: absence at birth, development during the life span, and dissolution in Alzheimer's disease, Ann Neurol 24(6):765-773, 1988.

Meyer JS et al: Improved cognition after control of risk factors for multi-infarct dementia, JAMA 256(16):2203-2209, 1981.

Meyer JS et al: Cognition and cerebral blood flow fluctuate together in multi-infarct dementia, Stroke 19(2):163-169, 1988.

Molsa PK, Marttila RJ, and Rinne UK: Survival and cause of death in Alzheimer's disease and multi-infarct dementia, Acta Neurol Scand 74:103-107, 1986.

Mortimer JA et al: Head injury as a risk factor for Alzheimer's disease, Neurology 35:264-267, 1985.

Moss MB et al: Differential patterns of memory loss among patients with Alzheimer's disease, Huntington's disease, and alcoholic Korsakoff's syndrome, Arch Neurol 43:239-246, 1986.

Mouradian MM et al: No response to high-dose muscarinic agonist therapy in Alzheimer's disease, Neurology 38(4):606-608, 1988.

Mufson EJ, Mash DC, and Hersh LB: Neurofibrillary tangles in cholinergic pedunculopontine neurons in Alzheimer's disease, Ann Neurol 24(5):623-629, 1988.

Nebes RD, Brady CB, and Jackson ST: The effect of semantic and syntactic structure on verbal memory in Alzheimer's disease, Brain Lang 36(2):301-313, 1989.

Nee LE et al: A family with histologically confirmed Alzheimer's disease, Arch Neurol 40:203-208, 1983.

Neshige R, Barrett G, and Shibasaki H: Auditory long latency event-related potentials in Alzheimer's disease and multi-infarct dementia, J Neurol Neurosurg Psychiatry 51(9):1120-1125, 1988.

Newhouse PA et al: Intravenous nicotine in Alzheimer's disease: a pilot study, Psychopharmacology 95(2):171-175, 1988.

Norbiato G et al: Alterations in vasopressin regulation in Alzheimer's disease, J Neurol Neurosurg Psychiatry 51(7):903-908, 1988.

Ogomori K et al: Beta-protein amyloid is widely distributed in the central nervous system of patients with Alzheimer's disease, Am J Pathol 134(2):243-251, 1989.

Olson CM: Vision-related problems may offer clues for earlier diagnosis of Alzheimer's disease [news] JAMA 261(9):1259, 1989.

Panella JJ et al: Day care for dementia patients: an analysis of a four-year progam, J Am Geriatr Soc 32:883-886, 1984.

Papasozomenos SC: Tau protein immunoreactivity in dementia of the Alzheimer type. I. Morphology, evolution, distribution, and pathogenetic implications, Lab Invest 60(1):123-137, 1989.

Parlato V et al: Patterns of verbal memory impairment in dementia. Alzheimer disease versus multinfarctual dementia, Acta Neurol (Napoli) 10(6):343-351, 1988.

Patterson JV, Michalewski HJ, and Starr A: Latency variability of the components of auditory event-related potentials to infrequent stimuli in aging, Alzheimer-type dementia, and depression, Electroencephalogr Clin Neurophysiol 71(6):450-460, 1988.

Peers MC et al: Cortical angiopathy in Alzheimer's disease: the formation of dystrophic perivascular neurites is related to the exudation of amyloid fibrils from the pathological vessels, Virchows Arch [A] 414(1):15-20, 1988.

Penn RD et al: Intraventricular bethanechol infusion for Alzheimer's disease: results of double-blind and escalating-dose trials, Neurology 38(2):219-222, 1988.

Perry E: Acetylcholine and Alzheimer's disease, Br J Psychiatry 152:737-740, 1988.

Peters CA, Potter JF, and Scholer SG: Hearing impairment as a predictor of cognitive decline in dementia, J Am Geriatr Soc 36(11):981-986, 1988.

Peterson C et al: Altered response of fibroblasts from aged and Alzheimer donors to drugs that elevate cytosolic free calcium, Neurobiol Aging 9(3):261-266, 1988.

Pettegrew JW et al: Correlation of phosphorus-31 magnetic resonance spectroscopy and morphologic findings in Alzheimer's disease, Arch Neurol 45(10):1093-1096, 1988.

Powers RE et al: Immunohistochemical study of neurons containing corticotropin-releasing factor in Alzheimer's disease, Synapse 1(5):405-410, 1987.

Prohovnik I et al: Cerebral perfusion as a diagnostic marker of early Alzheimer's disease, Neurology 38(6):931-937, 1988.

Prohovnik I et al: Gray-matter degeneration in presenile Alzheimer's disease, Ann Neurol 25(2):117-124, 1989.

Rai GS and Wright G: Tests for differential diagnosis of dementia of the Alzheimer's type, J Am Geriatr Soc 36(3):285, 1988 (letter).

Rasool CG, Svendsen CN, and Selkoe DJ: Neurofibrillary degeneration of cholinergic and noncholinergic neurons of the basal forebrain in Alzheimer's disease, Ann Neurol 20:482-488, 1986.

Rapcsak SZ et al: Lexical agraphia in Alzheimer's disease, Arch Neurol 46(1):65-68, 1989.

Reifler BV et al: Double-blind trial of imipramine in Alzheimer's disease patients with and without depression, Am J Psychiatry 146(1):45-49, 1989.

Represa A et al: Is senile dementia of the Alzheimer type associated with hippocampal plasticity? Brain Res 457(2):355-359, 1988.

Riisen H: Reduced prealbumin (transthyretin) in CSF of severely demented patients with Alzheimer's disease, Acta Neurol Scand 78(6):455-459, 1988.

Rinne JO et al: A comparison of brain choline acetyltransferase activity in Alzheimer's disease, multi-infarct dementia, and combined dementia, J Neural Transm 73(2):121-128, 1988.

Rocca WA, Amaducci LA, and Schoenberg BS: Epidemiology of clinically diagnosed Alzheimer's disease, Ann Neurol 19:415-424, 1986.

Rogers RL and Meyer JS: Computerized history and self-assessment questionnaire for diagnostic screening among patients with dementia, J Am Geriatr Soc 36(1):13-21, 1988.

Rosenberg RN et al: Dominantly inherited dementia and parkinsonism, with non-Alzheimer amyloid plaques: a new neurogenetic disorder, Ann Neurol 25 (2):152-158, 1989.

Rovner BW et al: Depression and Alzheimer's disease, Am J Psychiatry 146(3):350-353, 1989.

Roy BF et al: Antibody for nerve growth factor detected in patients with Alzheimer's disease, Ann N Y Acad Sci 540:398-400, 1988.

Sandman PO, Norberg A, and Adolfsson R: Verbal communication and behaviour during meals in five institutionalized patients with Alzheimer-type dementia, J Adv Nurs 13(5):571-578, 1988.

Schut LJ: Dementia following stroke, Clin Geriatr Med 4(4):767-784, 1988.

Seab JP et al: Quantitative NMR measurements of hippocampal atrophy in Alzheimer's disease, Magn Reson Med 8(2):200-208, 1988.

Seltzer B and Sherwin I: A comparison of clinical features in early- and late-onset primary degenerative dementia. One entity or two? Arch Neurol 40:143-146, 1983.

Shalat SL, Seltzer B, and Baker EL Jr: Occupational risk factors and Alzheimer's disease: a case control study, J Occup Med 30(12):934-936, 1988.

Sheridan PH et al: Relation of EEG alpha background to parietal lobe function in Alzheimer's disease as measured by positron emission tomography and psychometry, Neurology 38(5):747-750, 1988.

Shore D et al: Hair and serum copper, zinc, calcium, and magnesium concentrations in Alzheimer-type dementia, J Am Geriatr Soc 32:892-895, 1984.

Shuttleworth EC: Atypical presentations of dementia of the Alzheimer type, J Am Geriatr Soc 32:485-490, 1984.

Solomon PR, Beal MF, and Pendlebury WW: Age-related disruption of classical conditioning: a model systems approach to memory disorders, Neurobiol Aging 9(5-6):535-546, 1988.

Singh DN: Genes for Down syndrome and Alzheimer disease share the same chromosome 21, Indian J Pediatr 55(3):352-353, 1988.

Sirvio J et al: Cholinesterases in the cerebrospinal fluid, plasma, and erythrocytes of patients with Alzheimer's disease, J Neural Transm 75(2):119-127, 1989.

Smith FW et al: The use of technetium-99m-HM-PAO in the assessment of patients with dementia and other neuropsychiatric conditions, J Cereb Blood Flow Metab 8(6):S116-122, 1988.

Smith SR, Murdoch BE, and Chenery HJ: Semantic abilities in dementia of the Alzheimer type. 1. Lexical semantics, Brain Lang 36(2):314-324, 1989.

Soininen H et al: Treatment of Alzheimer's disease with a synthetic ACTH 4-9 analog, Neurology 35:1348-1351, 1985.

Sparks DL: Aging and Alzheimer's disease. Altered cortical serotonergic binding, Arch Neurol 46(2):138-140, 1989.

Stern Y, Sano M, and Mayeux R: Long-term administration of oral physostigmine in Alzheimer's disease, Neurology 38(12):1837-1841, 1988.

Stuart-Hamilton IA, Rabbitt PM, and Huddy A: The role of selective attention in the visuo-spatial memory of patients suffering from dementia of the Alzheimer type, Compr Gerontol [B] 2(3):129-134, 1988.

Summers WK et al: Oral tetrahydroaminoacridine in long-term treatment of senile dementia, Alzheimer type, N Engl J Med 315:1241-1245, 1986.

Sunderland T et al: A new scale for the assessment of depressed mood in demented patients, Am J Psychiatry 145(8):955-959, 1988.

Sunderland T, Tariot PN, and Newhouse PA: Differential responsivity of mood, behavior, and cognition to cholinergic agents in elderly neuropsychiatric populations, Brain Res 472(4):371-389, 1988.

Swearer JM et al: Troublesome and disruptive behaviors in dementia. Relationships to diagnosis and disease severity, J Am Geriatr Soc 36(9):784-790, 1988.

Tabaton M et al: Alz 50 recognizes abnormal filaments in Alzheimer's disease and progressive supranuclear palsy, Ann Neurol 24(3):407-413, 1988.

Talamo BR et al: Pathological changes in olfactory neurons in patients with Alzheimer's disease, Nature 337(6209):736-739, 1989

Tanaka S et al: Three types of amyloid protein precursor mRNA in human brain: their differential expression in Alzheimer's disease, Biochem Biophys Res Commun 157(2):472-479, 1988.

Tappen RM: Awareness of Alzheimer patients, Am J Public Health 78(8):987-988, 1988 (letter).

Tariot PN et al: Tranylcypromine compared with L-deprenyl in Alzheimer's disease, J Clin Psychopharmacol 8(1):23-27, 1988.

Tariot PN et al: High-dose naloxone in older normal subjects: implications for Alzheimer's disease, J Am Geriatr Soc 36(8):681-686, 1988.

Tariot PN et al: Multiple-dose arecoline infusions in Alzheimer's disease, Arch Gen Psychiatry 45(10):901-905, 1988.

Teri L et al: Behavioral disturbance, cognitive dysfunction, and functional skill. Prevalence and relationship in Alzheimer's disease, J Am Geriatr Soc 37(2):109-116, 1989.

Teri L, Larson EB, and Reifler BV: Behavioral disturbance in dementia of the Alzheimer's type, J Am Geriatr Soc 36(1):1-6, 1988.

Testa HJ et al: The use of [99mTc]-HM-PAO in the diagnosis of primary degenerative dementia, J Cereb Blood Flow Metab 8(6):S123-126, 1988.

Thal LJ, Grundman M, and Klauber MR: Dementia: characteristics of a referral population and factors associated with progression, Neurology 38(7):1083-1090, 1988.

Thal LJ et al: Chronic oral physostigmine without lecithin improves memory in Alzheimer's disease, J Am Geriatr Soc 37(1):42-48, 1989.

Thienhaus OJ et al: A controlled double-blind study of high dose dihydroergotoxine mesylate (Hydergine) in mild dementia, J Am Geriatr Soc 35:219-223, 1987.

Tierney MC et al: The NINCDS-ADRDA Work Group criteria for the clinical diagnosis of probable Alzheimer's disease: a clinicopathologic study of 57 cases, Neurology 38(3):359-364, 1988.

Trent B: Alzheimer's research: physicians begin to tread in an ethical minefield, Can Med Assoc J 140(6):726-728,730, 1989.

Tyson J: Portrait of an Alzheimer's patient: from masterful quilts to "mud pies" and toys, Nursing'88 18(12):36-37, 1988.

Urakami K, Adachi Y, and Takahashi K: A community-based study of parental age at the birth of patients with dementia of the Alzheimer type, Arch Neurol 46(1):38-39, 1989.

Vance DE, Ehmann WD, and Markesbery WR: Trace element imbalances in hair and nails of Alzheimer's disease patients, Neurotoxicology 9(2):197-208, 1988.

Vecsei L, and Widerlov E: Brain and CSF somatostatin concentrations in patients with psychiatric or neurological illness. An overview, Acta Psychiatr Scand 78(6): 657-667, 1988.

Waters C: Cognitive enhancing agents: current status in the treatment of Alzheimer's disease, Can J Neurol Sci 15(3):249-256, 1988.

Wenk GL: Amnesia and Alzheimer's disease: which neurotransmitter system is responsible? Neurobiol Aging 9(5-6):640-641, 1988.

Wilson RS, and Martin EM: New intrathecal drugs in Alzheimer's disease and psychometric testing, Ann N Y Acad Sci 531:180-186, 1988.

Wolozin BL et al: A neuronal antigen in the brains of Alzheimer patients, Science 232:648-650, 1986.

Wragg RE and Jeste DV: Neuroleptics and alternative treatments. Management of behavioral symptoms and psychosis in Alzheimer's disease and related conditions, Psychiatr Clin North Am 11(1):195-213, 1988.

Wright GM et al: Relationship between the P300 auditory event-related potential and automated psychometric tests, Gerontology 34(3):134-138, 1988.

Yamada M et al: Systemic amyloid deposition in old age and dementia of Alzheimer type: the relationship of brain amyloid to other amyloid, Acta Neuropathol (Berlin) 77(2):136-141, 1988.

Yamashita T et al: Detection of novel proteins associated with secondary amyloidosis and Alzheimer's disease by monoclonal antibody, Brain Res 474(2):309-315, 1988.

Yesavage JA: Nonpharmacologic treatments for memory losses with normal aging, Am J Psychiatry 142(5):600-605, 1985.

Zemlan FP, Thienhaus OJ, and Bosmann HB: Superoxide dismutase activity in Alzheimer's disease: possible mechanism for paired helical filament formation, Brain Res 476(1):160-162, 1989.

Zweig RM et al: A case of Alzheimer's disease and hippocampal sclerosis with normal cholinergic activity in basal forebrain, neocortex, and hippocampus. Part I, Neurology 39(2):288-290, 1989.

Glossary

abscess An accumulation of pus caused by infection.

abstracting ability The ability to shift voluntarily from one aspect of a situation to another. A characteristic of Alzheimer's disease and other psychiatric disorders is the inability to shift readily from the concrete to the abstract and back again as demanded by circumstances.

acetylcholine A neurotransmitter that is deficient in patients with Alzheimer's disease.

agnosia The inability to recognize various objects. Although agnosia often is present in early stages of Alzheimer's disease, it may be so subtle and slight that it goes unnoticed. In the early stages of Alzheimer's disease agnosia can be recognized only through detailed psychological tests.

amitriptyline (Elavil) A tricyclic antidepressant commonly given at bedtime. It has both sedative and anticholinergic side effects.

amnesia Memory impairment.

amyloid deposition Deposition of an abnormal protein (amyloid) in the brains of patients with Alzheimer's disease.

analgesics Medications used to relieve pain; painkillers.

angina See **Anginal pain.**

anginal pain The chest pain experienced by a patient with coronary artery disease. Typically this chest pain occurs during exercise and is relieved by rest or by appropriate medication. If such measures do not relieve the pain within a few minutes, the patient may have developed a myocardial infarction.

anomia Difficulty in finding the correct words for different objects. For example, the patient may recognize a pencil and may know what it is used for, but he or she will be unable to think of the word "pencil." Often the patient may use a sentence to describe a particular word. For instance, instead of "pencil," the patient may say "the thing you use to write with" or instead of "key," the patient may say "the thing used to open a door." Anomia is one of the first manifestations of Alzheimer's disease. Usually the patient first has difficulty naming objects he does not deal with in everyday life.

antacids Drugs given to reduce the acidity of the contents of the stomach.

antibiotics A group of drugs used to combat infection. For severe infections, antibiotics usually are administered intravenously; in most other cases, they are administered orally.

anticholinergic side effects Side effects produced by medication that inhibits the parasympathetic branch of the autonomic nervous system. These side effects include dry mouth, blurred vision, and urinary retention. Medications with anticholinergic side effects include antihistamines, neuroleptic drugs, and antidepressants. These drugs sometimes are combined with antacids.

antihistamines   Drugs taken for allergies and the common cold. Most antihistamines induce a certain degree of drowsiness and may cause sedation. They often are included in sleeping medications bought over the counter.

apathy   A condition in which the patient shows little or no emotion.

aphasia   An impairment in the speech process. "Receptive aphasia" is an inability to comprehend what one hears. "Expressive aphasia" is an inability to express oneself, even though the question has been heard and understood. The two types usually are differentiated by asking the patient to execute a certain command, such as closing eyes, sticking tongue out, or raising the left arm. If the patient hears and understands what is being said, he will execute the command. If he cannot hear or cannot comprehend what he hears (receptive aphasia), he will be unable to comply. When giving these commands, it is important not to mimic the gesture the patient is expected to perform. For instance, while asking the patient to raise his arm, the examiner must refrain from raising an arm.

apnea   Cessation of breathing. "Sleep apnea" is the cessation of breathing while sleeping, which characteristically occurs in grossly overweight and obese individuals. With apnea less oxygen reaches the brain, and the individual may wake up distressed.

apraxia   The inability to carry out purposeful movements and actions despite intact motor and sensory systems. Apraxia usually is present early in Alzheimer's disease but may be confined to actions the patient does not routinely perform during daily activities. For example, the patient may not be able to tie a bow tie, but may still be able to tie a regular tie; this is often attributed to a lack of practice. In early stages apraxia may be more manifest when the patient faces several choices. He may have no difficulty putting his shirt on, but when faced with a variety of shirts, ties, underwear, trousers, and coats, he may become confused as to which one to pick first. As the disease progresses, apraxia comes to affect even daily activities, and the patient no longer can dress, feed, or wash himself even though that he has no paralysis.

arteriosclerosis   A condition in which the inner lining of the arteries is coated with cholesterol, triglycerides and other fatty substances. This deposition, which often also invades other layers of an artery, causes the arteries to become rigid and their lumens narrow. This diminishes the amount of blood that flows through these arteries and the amount that reaches the various organs supplied by them. If arteriosclerosis affects the arteries taking blood to the brain, the blood supply to the brain is reduced and the patient is much more likely to develop a stroke.

aspiration pneumonia   A pneumonia caused by inhaling gastric contents or food into the lungs.

asthma   A disease in which the trachea and bronchi (airways) become constricted, reducing the amount of air reaching the lungs. Asthma characteristically occurs in attacks, with the patient experiencing sudden breathlessness and an inability to breathe comfortably. In many instances asthma reflects an allergic reaction to a number of substances that may contain pollen. Asthmatic attacks also are often precipitated by smoking.

atrophy   Wasting away. One of the characteristic features of Alzheimer's disease is the wasting away of the brain, which becomes much smaller than that of an individual of the same age and sex who does not have the disease.

autoanalysis   See **Biochemical screening.**

autonomic nervous system   The part of the nervous system that is not under voluntary control. The autonomic nervous system has two main subdivisions: the parasympathetic system and the sympathetic system. On the whole, the parasympathetic system takes over while a person is relaxing or sleeping, whereas the sympathetic system is predominantly active when an individual is in an excited state.

benzodiazepines   A class of drugs used to treat anxiety and insomnia. The group includes flurazepam (Dalmane), chlordiazepoxide (Librium), diazepam (Valium), and alprazolam (Xanax). Some patients become addicted to these drugs, and abrupt withdrawal may lead to seizures.

b.i.d.   (bis in die) An abbreviation designating that a medication be administered twice daily.

biochemical screening   A series of laboratory tests for measuring the concentration of various blood substances. The screening often is done on automated equipment and sometimes is referred to as autoanalysis or SMA (sequential multichannel autoanalysis).

bipolar disorder   A mood disorder comprising episodes of both mania and depression; formerly called "manic depressive illness." Patients with bipolar disorder may appear either manic or depressed.

bulimia   Episodic eating binges or excessive intake of food or fluid, generally beyond voluntary control. Although often a condition of young women, it is also seen in patients with Alzheimer's disease.

cachexia   Severe weight loss associated with dehydration.

calculi   (plural of *calculus*) Crystals or very small stones present in the urinary tract system. If a stone is present in the kidneys or ureters, the patient will have very severe flank pain radiating to the groin and will pass blood in the urine. If the stone is located in the urinary bladder the patient may feel a constant urge to empty the bladder, but only a few drops of urine are passed at a time. A bladder stone also is often associated with pain or scalding. When calculi are present in the bladder, they increase the excitability of the bladder and may be responsible for bouts of urinary incontinence.

cardiac reserve capacity   The heart's ability to increase its output to meet the body's increased demand during exercise.

cataract   A condition in which the lens of the eye becomes opaque. The condition is frequently seen in old age and is one of the most common causes of impaired visual acuity in older people. In some instances cataracts are caused by specific diseases such as diabetes mellitus, hyperparathyroidism, but most often the cause is unknown. Patients with cataracts often see better in dim light, because the pupils are dilated and a larger portion of the lens is exposed (in bright light, the pupils are constricted and only a small part of the lens is exposed). Cataract surgery is the treatment of choice.

cerebrovascular accident   See **Stroke.**

chlorpromazine (Thorazine)   A neuroleptic drug that belongs to the class of drugs known as phenothiazines. It causes extrapyramidal effects, sedation, and orthostatic hypotension.

cholesterol   A fatty substance present in the bloodstream that is essential for the adequate functioning of a number of body cells. However, if the concentration rises above a certain level, cholesterol tends to be precipitated along the inner lining of the arteries, giving rise to arteriosclerosis. This in turn is associated with an increased risk of developing coronary heart disease, strokes, and peripheral vascular insufficiency.

chromosomes   Microscopic, rod-shaped structures which are found in every living cell that contain a number of genes. The genes transmit the characteristics inherited from the parent cell to the next generation. It has been postulated that Alzheimer's disease may involve some defect in chromosome 21. This is the same chromosome that is defective in Down's syndrome and all patients with Down's syndrome who survive the third decade of life develop the manifestations of Alzheimer's disease.

circadian rhythm   See **Sleep/wake cycle.**

cognitive functions   The operations of the mind by which an individual becomes aware of objects of thought or perception. Includes all aspects of perceiving, thinking, and remembering.

congestive cardiac failure   A condition in which the heart cannot maintain an adequate output. The common manifestations of heart failure include swelling of the legs (particularly worse toward the end of the day) and breathlessness on exertion. One of the first signs is awakening several times a night to pass a large amount of urine. In early stages the patient tends to wake up in the middle of the night short of breath. This breathlessness usually is relieved when the patient sits up. In later stages the patient cannot lie flat in bed and must lie in a semisitting position supported by two, three, or four pillows.

coronary heart disease   A condition in which the lumina of the arteries supplying blood to the heart are narrowed by cholesterol deposition along their inner linings. Patients with coronary heart disease may have anginal pain or a myocardial infarct.

cortex   The outer layer of the brain. Alzheimer's disease affects the cortex: The number of brain cells (neurons) is reduced, and a number of typical microscopic findings can be seen, including neurofibrillary tangles and plaques.

computerized tomography (CT) scan   A special radiological test in which a very large number of x-ray films are taken simultaneously from different angles. The various pictures are put together by a computer to give a more detailed view of the brain. In advanced stages of Alzheimer's disease, the CT scan often reveals that the brain has atrophied and that the ventricles inside the brain are dilated. In early stages, however, the CT scan is essentially within normal limits. Although there has been a great deal of controversy over whether a CT scan should be done routinely in patients suspected of having Alzheimer's disease, the current consensus is that such an investigation is necessary. It must be emphasized, however, that this investigation is not necessary so much to confirm the diagnosis of Alzheimer's disease as to exclude other conditions that may mimic Alzheimer's disease, such as a brain tumor, brain hemorrhage, or stroke. A CT scan may be done with or without contrast medium. The former technique usually is preferred so that the various parts of the brain can be clearly visualized. The main problem with administering a CT scan is that the patient must lie still on the table, which is sometimes difficult for patients who have advanced Alzheimer's disease.

cross-sectional study   A study done at one point in time on several people of different ages. A number of these studies have been done in an attempt to examine the aging process, but it now is generally felt that most such studies can be misleading, because it is inaccurate to compare generation with generation and to attribute changes to the aging process when in fact most changes could be the result of changes in economic, cultural, and social circumstances. Currently, longitudinal studies are preferred, because they follow a group of individuals as they age. The main drawback of longitudinal studies is the long period before results become apparent, often exceeding 20 to 30 years. Two major longitudinal studies in progress are the Framingham study and the Baltimore study.

decubitus ulcer (plural is decubiti)   An ulcer that develops when a patient is bedridden for prolonged periods. The usual sites for these ulcers are the sacral region, the heels, and, in rare cases, the shoulder blades and the back of the head. To prevent decubiti, egg-crate mattresses or special beds should be used and the patients should be turned regularly while in bed.

delirium   An acute medical condition manifested by disorientation, confusion, and fluctuating levels of consciousness. Unlike Alzheimer's disease, delirium has an acute onset and is associated with semiconsciousness or an impaired state of consciousness. It usually is caused by a reversible condition.

delusions   False beliefs firmly held despite obvious proof or evidence to the contrary. These beliefs are not accepted by other members of the person's culture. Some examples are delusions of being controlled, delusions of grandeur (an exaggerated idea of one's own importance or identity), and delusions of persecution.

diabetes mellitus   A disease in which the body's utilization of glucose is reduced, resulting in an increase in the blood glucose level. Patients with diabetes mellitus often may experience acute confusion if the blood glucose level reaches a high level, or, if the condition is treated, if the blood glucose level is inadvertently reduced to a very low value.

diaphragm   The muscle that separates the chest from the abdominal cavity. The diaphragm plays an important role in breathing; by contracting and relaxing, it pulls on the chest wall, increases the volume of the chest, and facilitates the drawing of air into the lungs.

diazepam (Valium)   A benzodiazepine that is used to treat anxiety and muscle spasms. It is long acting and particularly liable to accumulate in elderly patients.

digitalis   A drug often used to treat heart failure, especially when the heart rate is irregular and rapid.

digoxin   See **Digitalis.**

diuretics   Drugs that increase the volume of urine produced. All diuretics increase the amount of sodium, as well as water, in the urine, and most also increase the amount of potassium lost in the urine. This may be particularly serious if the patient is simultaneously taking digitalis. The incidence of digitalis toxicity is increased if the patient has a low blood potassium level. Some diuretics also increase the amount of calcium lost in the urine.

diurnal pattern   See **Sleep/wake cycle.**

dysuria   Pain or a burning sensation while passing urine. Dysuria often denotes an infection in the bladder.

echolalia   The tendency to repeat a question asked or a word of a question without being able to answer the question.

electrocardiogram (ECG)   The graphic record of the heart's electrical activity. Electrocardiograms usually are obtained to detect insufficient blood supply to the heart or cardiac irregularities.

electroencephalogram (EEG)   The graphic record of the brain's electrical activity. In patients with Alzheimer's disease, the EEG shows that most brain waves are of smaller magnitude than those of normal individuals; generalized slowing may also be observed. Currently, an EEG is not necessary in the routine diagnostic workup of a patient suspected of having Alzheimer's disease.

electrolyte   A chemical substance in the blood. Examples include sodium, potassium, calcium, and magnesium. Electrolyte levels can be reduced or elevated by a number of diseases or by various medications.

embolism   The development of an embolus.

embolus   A clot or other blockage brought to a blood vessel from another part of the body.

endocrine disease   A disease of the endocrine or hormonal glands; including the thyroid, parathyroid, pituitary, and adrenals glands as well as the gonads.

estrogens   Hormones secreted by the ovaries. Estrogen secretion tends to decrease drastically during the menopause, and this sudden reduction may be responsible for a number of signs and symptoms, including atrophic vaginitis.

etiology   A technical term referring to the causes of a particular condition.

excoriation   A breaking down of the skin's surface, a condition associated with irritation. It often occurs when urine is left in contact with the skin.

extrapyramidal side effects (EPS)   A variety of signs and symptoms including muscular rigidity, tremors, drooling, shuffling gait, restlessness, peculiar involuntary posture, and motor inertia. Neuroleptic drugs are particularly liable to give rise to EPS.

flurazepam (Dalmane)   A hypnotic medication that tends to remain in the body for a long period, particularly in elderly patients. This may lead to drowsiness and unsteadiness the morning after the drug is taken.

genes   Microscopic structures located on the chromosomes that transmit specific characteristics from generation to generation.

Current studies in Alzheimer's disease are focusing on identifying a particular gene that may be defective. This would allow identification and accurate diagnosis of individuals with the disease and may in the future allow "repair" of the defective gene through genetic engineering. (See **Chromosomes**.)

genetic markers   Substances produced by abnormal genes; they can be found in individuals possessing these abnormal genes but not in people with normal genes.

genetic pattern   The organization and structure of various genes. It now is possible to identify abnormal genes in a number of diseases and to diagnose these diseases by finding the abnormal gene and abnormal genetic pattern.

glaucoma   A condition in which the fluid in the eye is under increased pressure. Glaucoma is a serious condition, since if allowed to persist, the pressure may interfere with the blood supply of the optic nerve and lead to blindness. A characteristic feature of glaucoma is the halos a patient often sees around objects; headaches also are common. Glaucoma can be managed relatively easily by administering eye drops regularly. Surgery also is sometimes used to treat this condition. In late stages, before vision is completely lost, the patient may have tunnel vision.

granulovacuolar degeneration   A microscopic finding describing degenerative changes in the brain cells.

gray matter   The structures in the brain that appear gray when the brain is cut; these include the outer layer of the cortex and a few structures in the center of the brain known as the basal ganglia. The gray matter contains most of the neurons.

gyri (plural of gyrus)   The convolutions seen on the surface of the brain. In Alzheimer's disease these tend to become narrower and less convoluted.

haloperidol (Haldol)   A neuroleptic drug that is one of the butyrophenones. It is a powerful medication with severe extrapyramidal side effects and should be given only for delusions, hallucinations, or bizarre behavior.

human immunodeficiency virus test (HIV)   A test performed to detect the virus responsible for acquired immunodeficiency syndrome (AIDS).

hyperthyroidism   A disease in which the thyroid gland is overactive. Patients with hyperthyroidism tend to be overactive and to feel as if they have an enormous amount of energy. They also tend to lose weight and to prefer cold weather.

hypnotics   Drugs that are given to induce sleep. Since drugs are metabolized more slowly as individuals age, the effect of hypnotics may be prolonged in an older individual, causing increased sleepiness. Also, older people may be more sensitive to these drugs.

hypothyroidism   A disease in which the thyroid gland does not produce sufficient thyroxin. Patients with hypothyroidism tend to tire easily, to become constipated, to sleep most of the time, and to be oversensitive to cold, preferring very warm environments.

illusion   A misperception of a real external stimulus, as when a shadow on the wall caused by the moon and a tree outside is perceived as a stranger entering the room.

imipramine (Tofranil)   A drug used to treat depression; it is one of the tricyclic antidepressants. Imipramine is particularly prone to causing anticholinergic side effects.

indwelling Foley catheter   A tube introduced through the urethra into the urinary bladder. A balloon at the end of the tube is inflated to keep the catheter in position. This type of catheter should be used only as a last resort in the treatment of urinary incontinence. Its use is associated with a number of side effects, most importantly urinary tract infections, which often spread from the bladder to the kidneys.

insight   A person's ability to be aware of his problems. In early stages of Alzheimer's disease, the patient usually has insight into his impaired mental functions, particularly his poor memory. As time passes and his condition deteriorates, this insight is gradually lost and he may not realize that he has a poor memory. Lack of insight is particularly useful in differentiating Alzheimer's disease from depression, which sometimes can give rise to apparently impaired mental functions, a condition referred to as "pseudodementia." In all but the early stage of Alzheimer's disease, the patient has no insight into his poor memory, whereas with depression the patient usually has this insight and often tends to exaggerate this memory problem. A depressed patient commonly will state that his memory is poor and thus he cannot remember what day of the week it is or cannot recall recent events. A patient with Alzheimer's disease, on the other hand, will maintain that his memory is quite good and readily confabulate, that is, give wrong answers about recent events or the day of the week.

intramuscular   A term denoting the route of administration of medication by injection into a muscle. The usual sites for intramuscular injection are the buttocks, thighs, and occasionally the shoulders.

intravenous (IV)   A term denoting the route of administration of medication or fluids when administered into a vein.

intravenous line   A slender tube that is inserted into a vein and kept in position to allow regular administration of medication or fluids.

Kegel exercises   A set of exercises designed to strengthen the pelvic floor and perineal muscles to control stress incontinence. These exercises consist mostly of constricting the external urinary sphincter and some of the perineal and pelvic muscles. The easiest way of knowing when these muscles contract is to attempt to interrupt the flow of urine while micturating. To be effective, Kegel exercises must be repeated as often as possible.

kyphoscoliosis   A condition in which the curvature of the thoracic vertebrae (the upper part of the back) is increased and is associated with a sideways deformity of the spine. This often is the result of osteoporosis.

kyphosis   A condition involving excessive curvature of the thoracic vertebrae. This often results from osteoporosis, because the increased fragility of the vertebrae causes them to become wedge shaped, thus increasing the normal curvature of the thoracic spine.

laxative   A drug taken to increase the bowel motions and to prevent constipation.

lipofuscin   A pigment that accumulates in the nerve cells as a person ages. It also accumulates in muscle, heart, and liver cells. The significance of this pigment is not fully understood.

lithium   Lithium carbonate is a salt used in the treatment of acute mania and as a maintenance medication to help reduce the duration, intensity, and frequency of recurrent episodes of bipolar disorder.

logoclonia   Repetition of the first syllable of a word the patient has just heard.

lumbar puncture   A test that involves introducing a needle through the back between two lumbar vertebrae to obtain a sample of the fluid (cerebrospinal fluid) that surrounds the spinal cord. Until recently a lumbar puncture was considered part of the routine diagnostic workup of patients suspected of having Alzheimer's disease, but it currently is not done routinely in these patients. It is reserved for the diagnosis of infections, tumors, multiple sclerosis, and other conditions affecting the spinal cord or brain.

magnetic resonance imaging (MRI)   A specialized radiological test that allows a clear view of various body organs. When done on the head, the brain can be clearly visualized. Although this test has become available, it is not yet used routinely in the diagnostic workup of patients suspected of having Alzheimer's disease.

metabolic diseases   Diseases that interfere with the body's metabolism. The concentration of various substances in the blood is maintained within a very narrow range of normality by a number of factors. For instance, glucose is controlled by the amount of insulin produced by the pancreas, in addition to a number of other factors. In metabolic diseases the concentration of these various substances is altered.

mood disorders   A group of disorders characterized by prominent and persistent disturbances in mood (depression or mania). The disorders usually are episodic but may be chronic.

morbidity   The state of being diseased.

mucosal smear   A test in which a few cells from the lining of the vagina (mucosa) are smeared on a glass slide and examined microscopically to determine whether enough estrogens (female hormones) are circulating in the blood. By examining these mucosal cells it is possible to tell whether a patient has atrophic vaginitis.

multiinfarct dementia   A condition in which the dementia is caused by repeated small strokes. Often these strokes do not give rise to any paralysis or other neurological deficit. However, as time goes by and more strokes are produced, gradually the number of brain cells diminishes and the patient may gradually manifest a dementing illness. It is important to differentiate multiinfarct dementia from

Alzheimer's disease, since the incidence of repeated strokes can be reduced and thus the progress of multiinfarct dementia sometimes can be stopped, leading to stabilization of the patient's condition. Unfortunately, with Alzheimer's disease progression of the disorder is usually relentless.

mutism A condition in which the patient does not communicate verbally with others.

myocardial infarction A condition that results when the blood flow through the coronary arteries taking blood to the heart is completely stopped. This usually happens when a blood clot develops in one of the coronary arteries, accompanied by complicating arteriosclerosis. The condition usually is manifested by severe central chest pain that is not relieved by either rest nor by sublingual nitroglycerin. The patient is apprehensive, usually sweating, and has a sense of impending death.

nasogastric tube A tube that is passed through the nasal cavity into the stomach. This tube usually is used to feed patients who have difficulty swallowing or who cannot feed themselves.

neoplasm A cancerous growth.

neurofibrillary tangles A microscopic finding in the neuron cells that is made up of aggregations of neurofilaments and neurotubules. These neurofibrillary tangles are commonly seen in normal aged brains but usually are few in number. In Alzheimer's disease, however, these tangles are widespread throughout the cortex and are quite dense.

neurofilament A slender filament present in the cells. Neurofilaments are thought to be involved in intracellular transport of metabolites.

neuroleptics Drugs used to treat psychotic symptoms. They include phenothiazines (e.g., Thorazine, Mellaril, Stelazine), butyrophenones (e.g., Haldol), and thioxanthenes (e.g., thiothixene or Navane).

neuromelanin A pigment inside the nerve cells.

neuron A nerve cell.

neurotransmitters Chemical substances that conduct electrical impulses from one cell to another and thus enable an electrical impulse to proceed. The main neurotransmitters that are deficient in Alzheimer's disease are acetylcholine, somatostantin, and to a lesser extent serotonin and dopamine.

nonsteroidal antiinflammatory compounds Medications given to patients with arthritis and other painful conditions. These drugs reduce inflammation and relieve pain. Common examples are aspirin and ibuprofen.

o.d. (omni die) An abbreviation designating that a medication be administered once a day.

oropharynx An anatomical term referring to the back of the mouth and upper part of the pharynx.

osteoarthritis A disease affecting the joints—particularly the hands, knees, and hips—that causes pain and stiffness. Characteristically the pain is much worse after exercise and tends to be somewhat relieved by rest. With osteoarthritis the cartilage lining the bones becomes less efficient at protecting the bones and preventing them from rubbing against each other in the joint. The cartilage gradually becomes frayed, and loose bits of cartilage may become dislodged in the joint. The exact cause of osteoarthritis is not known, although it currently is thought to be mostly a degenerative disease. It usually is treated with analgesics or nonsteroidal antiinflammatory drugs.

paralalia Repetition of the same words over and over.

paranoid disorders   Also called delusional disorders, these are mental conditions involving persistent delusions of persecution or jealousy; schizophrenia, mood disorders, and organic mental disorders have been excluded as causes in these cases.

parasympathetic nervous system   A division of the autonomic nervous system.

Parkinson's disease   A disease characterized by muscle stiffness and tremors; it is also known as "shaking palsy" or "shaking paralysis." The muscles are not weakened, but the tremors interfere with the patient's daily activities. Parkinson's disease is caused by damage to some parts of the brain (substantia nigra). Some patients with Parkinson's disease develop dementia, a condition often referred to as a subcortical dementia because the affected area of the brain lies below the cortex. The main biochemical abnormality in Parkinson's disease is a deficiency of the neurotransmitter dopamine. Many drugs can be used to treat Parkinson's disease.

peripheral vascular insufficiency   A disease in which the lumina of the arteries taking blood to the legs is considerably reduced. As a result the patient may develop intermittent pain in the leg muscles during exercise, but it usually is relieved by rest.

physostigmine   A chemical substance that decreases the breakdown of acetylcholine in the synapse.

pica   The craving and eating of unusual foods or other substances. Pica is seen in a variety of medical conditions, including Alzheimer's disease. Eating of paint, paper, or excessive amounts of ice is common.

positron emission tomography (PET scan)   A highly specialized test that reflects the metabolic activity of the brain. Currently it is not routinely available.

pressure areas   The areas of the body that are under pressure when an individual lies down, including sacral region, heels, shoulder blades, and back of the head. Patients who are immobile or bedridden for prolonged periods develop a decubitus ulcer.

pressure sore   See **Decubitus ulcer.**

progesterone   A hormone secreted by the ovaries; secretion tends to decrease dramatically during menopause.

prognosis   A forecast of what is likely to happen when an individual contracts a particular disease. In the case of Alzheimer's disease, the prognosis currently is bad because there is no effective cure and the disease is known to have a slow, progressive course. In general, the younger the individual when the disease manifests itself, the worse the prognosis.

prolapse   The displacement of an organ or part of an organ. Uterine prolapse denotes the displacement and descent of the uterus into the vagina; a bladder prolapse denotes the protrusion of the bladder into the vaginal wall. Both conditions are associated with urinary incontinence secondary to the altered normal architecture and relationship of the urinary bladder, uterus, and vagina.

promazine (Sparine)   A neuroleptic drug that is one of the phenothiazines. It is no longer widely used because of its sedative side effects.

prostatic hypertrophy   Enlargement of the prostate gland, a gland present in men at the junction of the bladder and the urethra. An enlarged prostate may compress the urethra and obstruct the flow of urine. When the pressure of urine in the bladder exceeds that of the sphincter, incontinence results; this type of incontinence is called overflow incontinence. Other signs of prostatic hypertrophy include difficulty in starting the flow of urine and a weak stream.

proton magnetic resonance   See **Magnetic Resonance Imaging.**

pseudodementia   A condition in which the patient shows impaired mental functions and dementia, but in which the underlying diagnosis is not dementia but depression.

psychoactive drugs   Drugs that affect the mind or behavior, such as antidepressant, anxiolytic, and neuroleptic medications.

psychological testing   A series of tests performed by psychologists to assess a patient's mental functions. These tests are described in the Appendix.

psychotropic drugs   Drugs that exert an effect on the mind and modify mental activity. (See **Psychoactive Drugs.**)

q.i.d. (quater in die)   An abbreviation designating that a medication be given four times a day.

respiratory reserve capacity   The ability of the respiratory system to increase its work to meet the body's increased demands during exercise.

rigidity, muscle rigidity   A condition in which the muscles become rigid and thus, movement becomes difficult. Muscle rigidity often is seen in patients with Parkinson's disease and in late stages of Alzheimer's disease. In the latter condition, the excessive rigidity causes the body to assume a generalized flexed position while the patient is lying in bed.

sacral plexus   An agglomeration of nerve fibers from the autonomic nervous system that is present in the sacral area. This part of the autonomic nervous system partly controls micturition.

sedatives   Medications used to calm a patient. They are particularly useful when a patient is agitated, irritable, and violent. They should not be used routinely in patients with Alzheimer's disease, since a major side effect is drowsiness, which may in turn worsen the patient's confusion.

senile macular degeneration   A degenerative condition of the retina that occurs in old age, and that causes diminished visual acuity and eventually blindness. Currently there is no satisfactory treatment.

senile plaque   A microscopic finding that describes a small mass between the neurons of the brain. Senile plaques are found in many older people but tend to be more numerous in patients with Alzheimer's disease.

sensory information   Information sent to the brain by one of the five senses (sight, hearing, touch, smell, and taste). For instance, when a person sees a pencil, the shape and appearance of the object are transmitted through the eye to the brain, where they are interpreted as a pencil. Similarly, when the ears detect a sound, this sensory information is transmitted to the brain, where it is interpreted and the individual becomes aware of the meaning of the sound. In late stages of Alzheimer's disease, the patient may not be able to recognize common objects or the people he lives with such as his spouse, children, or neighbors in a nursing home. This often leads the patient to accuse the spouse or neighbor of being an intruder, which is distressing to them.

septicemia   A condition in which an infection spreads to involve the blood. As a result of septicemia, bacteria or other infective organisms circulate in the bloodstream and may reach any organ.

serotonin   A neurotransmitter present in the brain. The concentration of serotonin usually is reduced in patients with Alzheimer's disease.

sleep apnea   See **Apnea.**

sleep/wake cycle   The 24-hour cycle during which individuals tend to sleep at night and remain awake during the day. This often is referred to as the "circadian rhythm" or "diurnal rhythm." Although the sleep/wake cycle mostly is related to the presence or absence of sunlight, it also is regulated by a number of hormonal glands, which secrete various hormones at different concentrations at various times of the day. These glands seem to be regulated by an internal clock. Interestingly, even when people are deprived of sunlight and timekeeping devices, they tend to retain a circadian sleep/wake cycle. Patients with Alzheimer's disease often have a disturbed sleep/wake cycle and tend to be awake and agitated at night and sleepy during the day. They often become particularly confused early in the evening, a phenomenon sometimes called the "sundown syndrome." The altered sleep/wake cycle is particularly stressful for caregivers and has been found to be the least tolerated symptom of Alzheimer's disease.

SMA 6, 18, or 29   See **Biochemical Screening.**

somatic complaints   Bodily symptoms such as headache, backache, and dizziness. These complaints may be caused by physical or emotional disorders.

stroke   A condition in which part of the brain is deprived of blood. This often is a complication of arteriosclerosis. The three common causes of strokes are (1) thrombosis, (2) embolism, and (3) hemorrhage. In older patients thrombosis is the most common cause and hemorrhage the least common.

subcortical dementia   A dementia caused by abnormalities in the areas of the brain lying below the cortex. In Alzheimer's disease the cortex (as well as some other areas below it) is grossly affected. In subcortical dementia the cortex is by and large spared, and it is the structures below it that are largely affected. A common example of subcortical dementia is that seen in some patients with Parkinson's disease.

sulci (plural of sulcus)   The fissures seen on the outer surface of the brain. In Alzheimer's disease these tend to become shallow.

sundown syndrome   A period of severe confusion, occasionally associated with agitation, irritability, and sometimes violence, that typically occurs toward the end of the evening. The cause of the syndrome is not well understood but probably is related to the concentrations of various hormones in the blood. It has also been suggested that this syndrome may stem from the reduced natural light at the end of the day, which may precipitate a confused state in the patient.

sympathetic nervous system   A division of the autonomic nervous system.

synapse   See **Synaptic Cleft.**

synaptic cleft   The space between two nerve cells. The electrical impulses generated in one nerve cell can pass across the synaptic cleft (synapse) by the release of chemical compounds known as neurotransmitters, which in effect transmit the electrical impulses from one nerve cell to the other.

thioridazine (Mellaril)   A neuroleptic drug that is one of the phenothiazines. Although it causes fewer extrapyramidal side effects than haloperidol, it produces far more sedation and orthostatic hypotension.

thrombosis   The development of a thrombus.

thrombus   A blood clot that forms inside a blood vessel. Often is precipitated by arteriosclerosis.

thyroid   A gland situated in the neck that secretes thyroid hormone. Should the secretion of thyroid hormone be excessive or insufficient, the patient may show a confusional state. Either imbalance also would worsen the degree of mental impairment seen in patients with Alzheimer's disease.

t.i.d. (ter in die)   An abbreviation designating that a particular medication is to be administered 3 times a day.

tranquilizers   Drugs intended to calm an individual without causing undue sedation. These drugs are better avoided or used sparingly in patients with Alzheimer's disease, as they tend to cause some drowsiness. Because elderly individuals cannot get rid of most drugs through their urine (or bile) as quickly and efficiently as younger people, repeated use of a tranquilizer or other drug may cause the medication to accumulate in the body and lead to drowsiness and even sedation.

triglyceride A fatty substance present in the blood that is essential for the proper functioning of many cells. As with cholesterol, if the concentration of triglycerides is excessive, arteriosclerosis may develop.

urethral stricture A constriction in the urethra that could lead to obstruction of the flow of urine and overflow incontinence.

urinary sphincters Two sphincters on the urethra; one is close to the junction of the urethra and the urinary bladder (the internal urinary sphincter), and the other is nearer the surface of the body (the external urinary sphincter). The external urinary sphincter can be contracted at will, and its main use is to postpone micturition for a short period of time. Normally urine is prevented from leaving the urinary bladder by the constant contraction of the internal urinary sphincter, which is controlled by the autonomic nervous system. The sympathetic division of this system causes the internal urinary sphincter to constrict, preventing the passage of urine; the parasympathetic component causes the internal sphincter to relax, encouraging voiding.

urinary stasis The presence of urine in the bladder after voiding (also called residual urine). This condition, which frequently is seen in men with prostatic hypertrophy, often invites infection.

urodynamic tests A series of tests that evaluate the relationship between the bladder, the urethra, and abdominal pressure to determine the cause of urinary incontinence.

venous return The blood returning from various parts of the body to the heart.

visual spatial skills Skills that enable an individual to integrate incoming information so that he can orient himself geographically and find his way about. These skills often are impaired in patients with Alzheimer's disease. One of the most common manifestations of this impairment is a tendency to become lost.

vital signs Pulse, temperature, blood pressure, and respiratory rate.

white matter A structure of the brain below the cortex that appears white when the brain is cut. White matter is made up mostly of nerve fibers that connect the neurons in the gray matter to other parts of the brain or the body.

Index

Overflow incontinence, 100-101
Oxygen in blood, Alzheimer's disease impacted by level of, 29-30

P

Pads
  absorbant, for urinary incontinence, 112
  protective, for urinary incontinence, 113-114
Pain, Alzheimer's disease affected by, 34
Paralalia, definition of, 8
Paranoid disorder, Alzheimer's disease differentiated from, 19
Paraphrasia, definition of, 7
Parkinson's disease
  basal ganglia affected by, 216
  dementia caused by, 13, 224
  falling as result of, 53
  stress incontinence related to, 99
Parties, Alzheimer's disease patient therapy with, 176
Paternalism, control of, in Alzheimer's disease patient care, 89
Patient; *see* Alzheimer's disease patient
Pelvic tumor, urinary obstruction caused by, 101
Performance sexuality, 80
Perineal muscles, weakness in, urinary incontinence caused by, 99
Pernicious anemia, vitamin B 12 deficiency as cause of, 75
Personality
  ability to cope with stress and, 134-135
  change in, dementia indicated by, 224
  testing of, dementia and, 237
PET; *see* Positron emission tomography
Pet therapy, 178-179
Phrenology, brain function described with, 212
Physical abuse of older adult, 145-146
Physical therapist, role of, 174-179
Physostigmine, Alzheimer's disease treated with, 46
Pica, danger of, to Alzheimer's disease patient, 57-58
Pituitary gland, function of, 217
Pleural effusion, reduction of blood oxygenation due to, 30
Pneumonia
  death caused by, 11
    in Alzheimer's disease patient, 14
  development of, in stage 3 Alzheimer's disease, 118

Pneumonia—cont'd
  prevention of, 172
  reduction in blood oxygenation due to, 30
Pneumothorax, reduction of blood oxygenation due to, 30
Pneumovaccine, pneumonia prevented with, 172
Poisoning, danger of, to Alzheimer's disease patient, 55
Polypharmacy
  avoidance of, 201
  multiple pathologies and, 199
Positron emission tomography, 213
  Alzheimer's disease diagnosis and, 24
Power of attorney, 189-190
  durable, 189
  need for, for Alzheimer's disease patient, 53
  regular, 189
Premarin; *see* Conjugate estrogen
Presenile dementia, definition of, 4
Principle of beneficence, definition of, 87
Principle of equity, definition of, 87
Principle of respect, definition of, 87
Privacy, lack of, sexuality affected by, 83
Problem solving ability, brain function and, 217
Progesterone, sleep affected by, 41
Progressive supranuclear palsy
  case study of, 230
  dementia caused by, 224
Prostate, cancer of, sexuality affected by, 82
Prostatic hypertrophy
  detrusor instability caused by, 100
  indications of, 106
  urinary obstruction caused by, 101
Prostatitis, sexual performance affected by, 82
Protein, recommended dietary allowance for, 74
Provera; *see* Medroxyprogesterone acetate
Prozac; *see* Fluoxetine
Pseudodementia
  arteriosclerosis as cause of, 20
  case study of, 233-234
  depression associated with, 224
PSNP; *see* Progressive supranuclear palsy
Psychoactive drugs, neurotransmitters affected by, 210
Psychological abuse of older adult, 145
Psychotropic drugs, abuse of Alzheimer's disease patient with, 145